Mlle Mehdia Gandi

Research on bionanocomposites with therapeutic properties

Mlle Mehdia Gandi

Research on bionanocomposites with therapeutic properties

Fourth Edition

ScienciaScripts

Imprint

Any brand names and product names mentioned in this book are subject to trademark, brand or patent protection and are trademarks or registered trademarks of their respective holders. The use of brand names, product names, common names, trade names, product descriptions etc. even without a particular marking in this work is in no way to be construed to mean that such names may be regarded as unrestricted in respect of trademark and brand protection legislation and could thus be used by anyone.

Cover image: www.ingimage.com

This book is a translation from the original published under ISBN 978-620-6-72804-7.

Publisher:
Sciencia Scripts
is a trademark of
Dodo Books Indian Ocean Ltd. and OmniScriptum S.R.L publishing group

120 High Road, East Finchley, London, N2 9ED, United Kingdom
Str. Armeneasca 28/1, office 1, Chisinau MD-2012, Republic of Moldova, Europe
Printed at: see last page
ISBN: 978-620-0-07751-6

Table of contents

Part 1: Bibliographic research

GENERAL INTRODUCTION

Chitosan (CS), a linear biopolymer abundant in nature and inexpensive compared to others, its particular cationic nature in acidic environments, and its chelating power, make it a material of choice in the manufacture of bionanocomposites.

Bionanocomposites can be classified according to three parameters: consistency, the nature of the chemical bonds, and the origin of the materials.

There are three categories of CS-based bionanocomposites, depending on their consistency: particles, films and scaffolds. There are various processes for making them, but generally speaking, particles are manufactured by supramolecular complexation or ionotropic gelation; films by evaporation of dilute CS solutions; and scaffolds (for drug or medical devices) by freeze-drying.

In this research we focused on CS particles or, more precisely, CS bionanocomposite hydrogels. Firstly, and in the absence of a syringe pump (or dosing pump, a device used in ionotropic gelation), we attempted to formulate a CS bionanocomposite hydrogel that is physical and not chemical, bearing in mind that CS bionanocomposites in the form of chemical hydrogels can be made by adding a chemical binder in the absence of a dosing pump.

The second categorization parameter depends on the nature of the chemical bonds in these bionanocomposites: either they are weak and thus called physical bionanocomposite hydrogels (also semi-interpenetrating or supramolecular), in which case supramolecular complexation will govern the preparation reaction, or they are strong and covalent and thus called chemical bionanocomposite hydrogels.

The third criterion for differentiating bionanocomposites, in the general case, is the origin of the materials making up the composite mixture: either mineral, organic or ceramic.

On the other hand, visual and tactile analysis in the pharmaceutical industry is essential for pre-formulation and the design of galenic formulas, as well as for in-process inspection. It improves drug appearance and consistency, as well as homogeneity.

Chapter 1: Chitosan, a material for the preparation of bionanocomposites.

I.1.1. General information on Chitosan :

Chitosan is a macromolecule, often considered biocompatible, belonging to the family of complex sugars and carbohydrates. Its relatively affordable price, its cationic ionized structure and its chelating role make it stand out. Its two main characteristics are its degree of deacetylation (DD%) and its molecular weight.

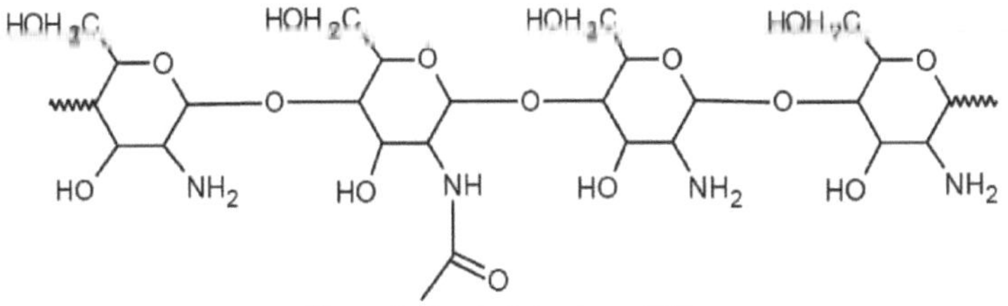

Figure 1. chemical structure of CS.

1.1.2. The therapeutic properties of Chitosan :

CS has a certain cytotoxicity, despite its usefulness in curing infections, inflammations and skin cancers. It has excellent muco-adhesive properties. It is also a vector for the controlled release of active drug ingredients.

1.1.3. Definition of Hydrogel as a Bionanocomposite :

Hydrogel is a composite because it is made up of two phases, a liquid phase held together by a solid phase. It is a nanocomposite because of the presence of silver or chitosan antiseptic metallic fillers, on a nanometric scale (100-1000 nm), and a bionanocomposite thanks to the chitosan biopolymer.

1.1.4. Main criteria for hydrogels

- **Depending on polarity**, there are two types: **hydrophilic** (hygroscopic) and **lipophilic**.
- **According to the nature of the chemical bonds**: **physical** (supramolecular, or semi-interpenetrated), and **chemical** (covalent bonds).
- **Depending on route of administration**: **oral** and **topical** or **injectable** (transdermal).
- **According to therapeutic effect**: **antiseptic, analgesic, anti-inflammatory, antibiotic, laxative.**

1.1.5. The Most Popular Gelling Agents for Chitosan Hydrogels

Physical gelling agents (they make highly physical gels): polyoxyethylene and polyethylene glycol.

Chemical gelling agents (they make weakly physical gels - in reality, it's a concept misclassified in the past, in the absence of more pragmatic processes, contemporary resistant hydrogels): beta glycerophosphate, tween 80, sodium tripolyphosphate and alginate.

Chapter 2: Silver, an effective antiseptic.

I.2. Silver, an effective antiseptic agent

The ability of silver nanoparticles (reinforcement) to be protected by chitosan (matrix) synergizes the antiseptic efficacy of chitosan-agent nitrate bionanocomposite hydrogels, at lower cytotoxicity. Chapters 3, 4, 5 and the conclusion contain bibliographical and experimental research on Ag NPs. This second chapter is the briefest in the thesis, in order to understand the primary objective of using the substrates in this study to synthesize an antiseptic hydrogel for topical application. This hydrogel is also an anti-inflammatory, as inflammations are often linked to an aggression such as an injury or an infection.

Chapter 3: Acetic acid as a polymerization initiator for chitosan bionanocomposites.

Introduction Chapter 3

The first systematic study of the solubility of chitin and CS was carried out by Austin, who introduced the solubility parameters of chitin in various solvents (Pillai, 2009). With three reactive groups, CS is more chemically active than chitin. Its reactive groups are primary and secondary hydroxyl groups in each repeat unit and an amino group on each deacetylated unit (Liu, 2011). The amino groups of CS are much easier to cationize and adsorb anions strongly by electrostatic attraction (Chiou, 2004). A number of studies have been carried out on this polymer, both on its cationic property, which stimulates cross-linking with materials of opposite charge, and on its solubility in acidic solutions (Austin et al.1977 & 1984; Demarger et al, 1994; le Dung et al., 1994; Rinaudo et al., 1999; Chiou et al., 2004; Huang et al., 2004; Pillai et al., 2009; Nallamuthu et al., 2014; Zain et al., 2014; Li et al., 2015; Kozicki et al., 2016; Jovanovic et al., 2016; Furuike et al., 2017). As for the choice of a solvent for CS characterization, different systems have been proposed, including an acid at a given concentration for protonation with a salt to screen electrostatic interaction (Rinaudo et al., 2006). We have tried to detail several previous researches important for this subject, then we have explained in a simplistic way, what happens at the monomer level when the CS is dissolved in an aqueous solution of a weak acid, more precisely the 1% acetic acid solution (below pH 6), at ambient temperature and pressure; and with a specific technique if we want to obtain Nano CS in the suspension. On the other hand, we have not shown the inter-chain H-bonds (involving the CS hydroxyl groups (Rinaudo, 2006)), in the reaction mechanism schemes, as they have always been recognized for their weaknesses.

1.3.1. **Bibliographic research**

1.3.1.1. **A few basics you need to know about Chapter 3**

The methods used to determine the solubility parameter are the group contribution method (GCM), maximum intrinsic viscosity, surface tension, Flory-Huggins interaction parameter and dielectric constant values. For each solvent system, a number of parameters such as polymer concentration, pH, counterion concentration, temperature effect, molecular weight, DD%, CS (Pillai, 2009), the distribution of acetyl groups along the chain (random or clockwise, as they are hydrophobic due to methyl functions) and the nature of the acid used for protonation (Rinaudo, 2006), are known to influence the dissolution process and solution viscosity. Dissolution may involve several days of penetration and swelling before solution (Pillai, 2009). With regard to the insolubility of CS, it has been found that the critical value of its DA for reaching insolubility in acidic media is above 60% (meaning that CS is poorly soluble in the DA range between 50% and 60%). Moreover, solubility at neutral pH has also been claimed for CS with DA of around 50%. A water-soluble form of CS at neutral pH was obtained in the presence of glycerol 2-phosphate. Stable solutions were obtained at pH 7-7.1 and at room temperature, but a gel formed on heating to around 40°C. The solgel transition was partially reversible and the gelation temperature was slightly dependent on experimental conditions (Rinaudo, 2006). As in the case of cellulose, the existence of intra- and intermolecular hydrogen bonds for chitin and CS in the solid state strongly resists dissolution. Due to the semi-crystalline structure of CS with extensive hydrogen bonding, the cohesive energy density will be high and therefore the solubility parameter will be low, tending to render CS insoluble in all the usual solvents. Many of the solvents previously used were toxic, corrosive, degrading or mutagenic, and so could not be used in medical applications, and also had difficulty in being developed for industrial production. In many cases, the solvents were strong acids, fluorinated alcohols, chloroalcohols and certain hydrotropic salt solutions, which either degraded chitin and therefore CS, or were impractical to use. Organic acids such as acetic, formic and lactic acids can dissolve CS, but it is also insoluble in sulfuric, phosphoric and other organic acids such as dimethylformamide and dimethylsulfoxide.

The best solvent for CS is formic acid (FA). But the most commonly used solvent is 1% acetic acid (as a reference) at around pH 4.0. Concentrated acetic acid solutions at high temperatures can cause depolymerization of CS (Pillai, 2009). However, modifying CS at the molecular level increases its solubility and stability, making it more versatile as a biopolymer (Cheung, 2015). CS is a water-soluble cationic derivative only when pH $\leq$ 6. It is of interest to prepare a cationic derivative that is readily soluble over the entire pH range. CS can readily form quaternary nitrogen salts at low pHs, but only when dissolved in concentrated strong acids, at above standard temperature ($\approx$ 60 ° C) and in the presence of concentrated sodium hydroxide solution ($\approx$ 15% by weight). Increasing the sodium hydroxide concentration leads to an increase in the degree of quaternization and an increase in the molecular weight of the CS as well, but partial polymer degradation may occur (le Dung, 1994).

While chitin is insoluble in most organic solvents, CS is readily soluble in dilute acid solutions below pH 6.0. Indeed, CS can be considered a weak base, as it possesses primary amino groups with a pKa value of 6.3. The presence of amino groups indicates that pH significantly alters the charged state and properties of CS. At low pH, these amines protonate and become positively charged, making CS a water-soluble cationic polyeletrolyte. On the other hand, as pH rises above 6, the CS amines become deprotonated and the polymer loses its charge and becomes insoluble. The soluble-insoluble transition occurs, with its pKa value around pH between 6 and 6.5. The pKa value of CS is highly dependent on the degree of N-acetylation, while the solubility of CS depends on the DD in addition to the deacetylation method used (Pillai, 2009). Conversion of chitin to CS can be achieved by enzymatic or chemical deacetylation. Chemical deacetylation is more commonly used for commercial preparation due to economic issues and the feasibility of mass production (Cheung, 2015). Solubility also depends on ionic concentration. The amount of acid required is known to depend on the amount of CS to be dissolved. The concentration of protons required is at least equal to the concentration of -NH2 units involved. Solubility is therefore a very difficult parameter to control, as it involves a complex set of controlling factors. In addition to DD, molecular weight is also an important parameter that significantly controls solubility and other properties (Pillai, 2009). Variations in CS molecular weight are controlled by the measurement of intrinsic viscosity, as there is an established proportional relationship between these two physical parameters (le Dung, 1994). Acetic acid is defined as a weak acid (Bleam, 2017), whereas, for example, HCl is considered a strong acid (Clegg, 1986) (which is why it is rarely used as a CS pharmacogelator stimulator). Hydrogen bonding is an electrostatic attraction between hydrogens and polar molecules, at nitrogen or oxygen atoms (the latter as in CS). These bonds are not so strong that they cannot be cut, but strong enough not to be cut easily (Makishima, 2017). This is why HCl was easier compared to CS, to cut intra/interchain CS H bonds, to remove primary and secondary hydroxyl groups from CS (Bleam et al., 2017; Clegg et al., 1986; Makishima et al., 2017). Rinaudo et al. (1999) studied the protonation of CS. It was studied in acetic acid and aqueous hydrochloric solutions with different

concentrations of acid or polymer. All measurements were carried out at 25 ±
0.1°C. The degree of protonation was determined and its variation with CS
concentration was established. The degree of protonation increases
progressively with CS solubilization. CS in acid medium becomes a
polyelectrolyte due to protonation of the -NH2 groups according to the equation
below (Rinaudo, 1999):

$$CS - NH_2 + H_3O^+ \leftrightarrow CS - NH_3^+ + H_2O$$

$$K_n = \frac{[CS - NH_2]\,[H_3O^+]}{[CS - NH_3^+]}$$

Examination of the role of CS protonation in the presence of acetic acid and
hydrochloric acid on solubility has shown that the degree of ionization depends
on the pH and pK of the acid. Solubilization of CS with low DA occurs for an
average degree of ionization α of CS around 0.5; in HCl, $\alpha = 0.5$ corresponds to
a pH of 4.5-5. Solubility also depends on ionic concentration, and a release
effect was observed in excess of HCl (1 M), enabling the hydrochloride form of
CS to be prepared. When the hydrochloride and acetate forms of CS are isolated,
they are directly soluble in water giving an acidic solution with pK0 = 6 ± 0.1,
in agreement with previous data and corresponding to the extrapolation of pK
for a degree of protonation $\alpha = 0$, so CS is soluble at pH below 6 (Rinaudo,
2006). It was also observed in these experiments that the concentration of acetic
acid must be 60% relative to that of CS to achieve solubility. After a comparison
between HCl and acetic acid for the same initial polymer concentration in
aqueous acid media (7.46 × 10⁻3) mol / l), we found that the viscosity of the
solutions increased at a higher rate and more rapidly in the presence of CH3COOH,
whereas it was, slightly and slowly reduced by HCl. Solubility was observed in
16.5 M acetic acid (the amount of CS to be dissolved was relatively large)
(Rinaudo, 1999).

I.3.1.2. **Spheres CS - TPP as adsorbent for anionic dyes**

Since high adsorption potentials for anionic dyes, metal ions, proteins and others
have been observed in CS, Chiou et al. (2004) investigate the equilibrium and
adsorption dynamics of eight anionic dyes on chemically cross-linked CS beads

in the pH range 3-8. CS contains high levels of amino functional groups, which could form an electrostatic attraction between CS and solutes to adsorb dyes and proteins. The binding capacity of CS for metal ion is also and mainly due to the chelating groups (amino and hydroxyl groups) on CS. To prepare the CS beads, they were first dissolved in acetic acid, which is often used as a stimulator in the staining process. To this end, ten grams of CS (type α; extracted from snow crab shell, degree of deacetylation: 95.5%; average molecular weight: 200 kD) were dissolved in 300 cm^3 , 5% by weight of an acetic acid solution. The aqueous solution was diluted to 1.0 dm^3 by vigorous agitation overnight, then left to stand still for 6 h. A solution of CS (10 cm^3) was poured from the burette, into a 100 cm^3 aqueous solution of TPP (purity $\geq$ 98%; 1% by weight) and formed beads with diameters of 2.3-2.5 mm, this is ionotropic gelation. TPP was used in the bead formation step to produce stiffer beads via its ionic cross-linking effect. The ionically cross-linked CS beads were washed with deionized water and stored in distilled water.

The above ionically cross-linked CS beads, 50 cm^3 of 1 N sodium hydroxide solution and the chemical cross-linking reagent ECH (purity $\geq$98%, a chemical cross-linking reagent, which was used to cross-link CS beads under alkaline conditions) were mixed and stirred for 6 h at 50°C in a water bath. The 0.5% molar ratio of cross-linking reagents to CS was achieved in this work. The ionic interaction between CS and TPP disappeared due to deprotonation of the adsorbent by 1 N sodium hydroxide prior to the chemical cross-linking reaction taking place in basic solution. In these experiments, CS beads chemically cross-linked (presence of ECH) were insoluble in acidic solutions of pH 3, while those not chemically cross-linked dissolved in acidic solutions below pH 5.5. The mixture of CS beads (containing 0.1 g dry CS base), dye solution (50 cm^3) and acetic acid buffer solution with the desired pH value were stirred for 5 days using a bath to control the temperature at 30 $\pm$ 1°C . Adsorption capacity increased slightly with decreasing CS bead diameter, since the effective surface area was higher for the same mass of smaller particles. This may suggest that adsorption took place mainly on the outer surfaces of the particles, due to the steric hindrance of large dye molecules. Thus, beads with diameters of 2.3-2.5 mm were used in this work to achieve a higher adsorption capacity. Cross-linked CS beads had very high adsorption capacities for removing anionic dyes. The major adsorption site for CS was the amine group -

NH2, which is readily protonated to form - NH3+ from CS and dye anions were used to explain the high adsorption capacity of anionic molecules on chemically cross-linked CS beads. At lower pH, more protons were available to protonate the amine groups of CS molecules to form -NH3+ groups, thus increasing electrostatic attractions between negatively charged dye anions and positively charged adsorption sites and causing increased dye adsorption. Chitin contains an amide group, -CO- NH-, which cannot be easily protonated in acidic solutions. Since the removal of electrons by the carbonyl group makes the nitrogen of the amide group a much poorer source of electrons than that of the primary amine group. Electrons are less available to be shared with a hydrogen ion, and so the amide is a much weaker base than the amine. The low adsorption capacity of chitin was due to the absence of electrostatic interaction between chitin and dye anions (fewer amines). It was reported that its main adsorption site was neither -OH nor -CH2OH, for which chitin and CS had the same amount. After a comparative study, CS appears to be much more effective than commercial activated carbon and chitin for color adsorption in the removal of anionic dyes, which can be projected onto the adsorption of anionic toxins in the human body (Chiou, 2004).

I.3.1.3. **CS-NaOH hydrogel as a cost-effective method for CS solubilization**

Furuike et al. (2017) noted that the solubility of CS (with DD: 84.7%) was remarkably improved by hydrogelation, as demonstrated by the small amount of acid required for dissolution compared with CS powder. The CS hydrogel was easily prepared by adding sodium hydroxide solution to CS acetic acid solution. Only 0.4 equivalents of the carboxyl group were required to neutralize one sugar unit of CS in the hydrogel. Since the degree of deacetylation of CS used in this study was around 80%, only 0.5 molar equivalents of anions were sufficient to neutralize one amino group of CS and dissolve the CS hydrogel. This result implies that acids can easily penetrate between CS molecules as the CS crystal structure has been destroyed under hydrogel conditions and a large amount of water molecules exist around the CS molecules. On the other hand, the viscosity of CS powder solutions has decreased considerably compared to CS hydrogel, since after 7 days it has decreased by 60%. To investigate changes in the viscosity of CS solutions, CS hydrogel or CS powder were dissolved in 0.1 M acetic acid, and the pH was adjusted to 3 and 5. The concentrations of the CS solutions obtained were 0.5 g dL^{-1} . These solutions were stored for 0 to 168 h. Finally, the viscometer was used for measurements on several occasions, and given the results obtained, we deduced that the preparation of CS solutions from CS hydrogels is preferred to inhibit the decrease in CS molecular weight (Furuike, 2017).

I.3.1.4. **Dissolution of CS in acetic acid for deacetylation**

Very low DA chitosans were rarely prepared due to the difficulty of deacetylation and the risk of degradation. We have previously obtained this polymer after three successive treatments in the presence of organic solvents (le Dung, 1994). This was followed by industrial deacetylation using highly concentrated hydroxides (40-50%). In 1993, Rinaudo patented a new deacetylation method using aqueous sodium hydroxide (5 or 10% by weight). This was the first deacetylation method to induce less polymer degradation, while at the same time generating an almost fully deacetylated derivative that was completely soluble in acetic acid. In this process, the starting material was first purified by solubilization in acetic acid (pH 4.5), filtered and then reneutralized with NH4OH, the flocculated polymer was recovered by filtration, washed and dried at room temperature (25°C). The purified CS was then dissolved in acetic acid, heated to a given temperature (100°C) and poured into the NaOH solution containing: thiophenol (1 ml / g CS), or NaBH4 (0.1 g / g CS)), or both; the role of these additives is to reduce polymer degradation, they are antioxidants. Experiments have shown that only a 5% NaOH solution enables deacetylation. The parameters that influenced deacetylation at constant temperature (100°C) were polymer concentration, reaction time and the presence of additives used to reduce polymer degradation. The chitosans obtained were characterized by their degree of acetylation, in D2O / CD3COOD by H NMR[1] , and their intrinsic viscosities were measured in CH3COOH 0.1 N / NaCl 0.2 N at 25°C as done by Roberts et al. (1982). The properties of the initial polymer (CS) were DA = 11% and $[\eta]$ = 1020 ml / g, and the smallest DA found was 2%, in 10% aqueous NaOH without any addition of antioxidants, it also had the lowest intrinsic viscosity 470 ml / g (so the molecular weight decreased significantly), while deacetylation lasted 5 h. Although we wanted to achieve the minimum DA, a reduction in reaction time also allows for a reduction in polymer degradation. For this reason, 5% aqueous NaOH, to which only NaBH4 was added, was the best deacetylation solution, as it had the shortest reaction time (3 h), even the DA obtained with the use of this solution was lower than 5%, it was only 3 ± 1%, and for which the viscosity remained almost stable (940 ml / g), so the molecular weight was not greatly affected (le Dung, 1994). In

Rinaudo's analyses, the H signal[1] was attributed to deacetylated units and its position depended on protonation. In the NMR spectrum, the degree of acetylation is determined from the integral of the CH3 peak of the acetyl group. We found that the degree of acetylation determined from the CH3 signal of the acetyl substituent was generally lower when HCl (7.4%) is used to solubilize CS, compared to acetic acid, due to the lower resolution of peaks attributed to acetyl groups (Liu, 2011). Thus, in addition, it has also been established that the acid used for CS solubilization prior to deacetylation in NaOH, affects DA values, as the pH changes and this can alter CS solubility and chemical shifts (le Dung, 1994).

1.3.1.5. The nature of CS/ CH3COOH interactions

In 1993, Demarger et al. studied the combination of CS and various carboxylic acids, namely formic, acetic, butyric and valeric acid in solutions and films. Due to the β- (1→ 4) bonds between the residues making up the chain, CS has good film-forming and fibrous properties, leading to a significant proportion of its applications. Films are easily obtained by evaporating dilute acid solutions of the polymer. It therefore seemed worthwhile to characterize the acid-base properties of CS in relation to the stability of films formed with different acids. Interactions occurring in aqueous solutions were characterized by potentiometry (pH-metry), while Fourier transform infrared spectroscopy (FTir) and X-ray diffraction were used to analyze solid materials and more specifically their evolution over time. All aqueous solutions of the acids studied were prepared and titrated with NaOH. CS was then dissolved in a stoichiometric quantity of a given acid, to form the corresponding CS salt solution of 0.5 mM concentration. Films were obtained by spreading such solutions on glass microscope slides and drying them in air or vacuum at 70°C for 15 min, then storing them for 6 months, with no special treatment required. Demarger et al. neutralized the CS / carboxylic acid solutions by NaOH titration, to determine the nature of the interactions existing between the two components. Next, pH was measured as a function of α, the dissociation coefficient of the ammonium function -NH3+. A comparison was made in the NaOH titration, between the different equimolar CS/ carboxylic acid solutions and the CS hydrochloric solution, as it was known that the latter acid exhibits a purely electrostatic interaction with CS. The curves representing the evolution of pH as a function of α, were similar and in particular had the same equivalent point, close to 7.1. Thus, Demarger et al. deduced that the interactions between CS and the various carboxylic acids were therefore of the same type occurring in the case of hydrochloric acid, implying that they are purely electrostatic. These results contradicted the reports of Sakurai et al. 1984, who stated that CS formed a true complex with butyric acid. After neutralization with NaOH and addition of CS, a variation in the initial pH (pHi) of the solutions was observed, which is largely dependent on the counterions. We found that the pHi of the solution was directly related to the pKa of the corresponding carboxylic acid. In the case of butyric and valeric acid salts, the concentration of H + ions was respectively around three and five times lower than that of formic and hydrochloric acids. Remember that the pK0 of CS is close to 6.5. This means that the amino function of CS is a weak base and that we are therefore in their case typically in the presence of salts corresponding to weak acids (even acetic acid is one of them (Bleam, 2017)) and a weak base. Their aqueous salts are only partially formed and in equilibrium with a significant proportion of the acids remaining in undissociated form. This is of great interest for biological applications, as thanks to them, CS would be considered as an acid carrier for sustained-release acid delivery systems. This has led to numerous applications in the fields of cosmetics, wound healing and dietetics. Since the counterion affects the apparent pKa of CS salts, the pH of these solutions can be raised to 5 or more, simply by partial protonation of the polysaccharide with butyric, acetic and valeric acids (undesirable reactions in biological media due to the acidity of some CS, can thus be minimized). FTir analysis of CS films confirmed the purely electrostatic nature of the relationship between CS and the various carboxylic acids. The second observation, based on the FTir results, concerns the drying of CS carboxylate films. As the films dried, the CS -NH3+ and carboxylic acid -COO⁻ bands progressively regressed. In the case of acetic acid, all the acid's IR absorption bands disappeared after 6 months, and the FTir spectrum obtained was identical to that of pure CS in its free amine form. In contrast, in the case of CS butyrate and CS valerate films, the loss of acid content remains incomplete even after 6 months of drying. This can be attributed to their boiling points above the boiling point of acetic acid ($\approx 118°C$, 165°C and 187°C for acetic, butyric and valeric acids respectively) and the low solubility of acetic acid in water. A second important parameter was the solubility of carboxylic acid, which decreased rapidly with increasing molecular weight of CS films. In contrast to freshly prepared films, all 6-month-old CS carboxylate films became insoluble in pure water. Whatever the drying time, CS hydrochloride films remain soluble, as their chemical structure remains unchanged during drying. This must be linked to the fact that, in the case of weak acids, the CS -NH3+ content decreases considerably during drying, and the proportion of the -NH2 form, which is thus regenerated, is sufficient to induce CS insolubility. We set the insolubility limit for the proportion of regenerated -NH2 function at over 45% (for CS obtained from totally deacetylated chitin using a method developed by Domard and Rinaudo (1983) (Demarger, 1994).

I.3.1.6. **Some important facts about CS-based gelation**

It has been reported that at higher pH, precipitation or gelation of the CS-acid solution tends to occur. Thus, the concentration of the acid plays a major role in conferring the desired functionality (Pillai, 2009). On the other hand, we have found that microcrystalline CS can be a gel-forming excipient. Matrix granules of CS with different physico-chemical properties loaded with active substances as drug models have been prepared for several years. Drug release from CS-based particle systems depends on the extent of cross-linking, the morphology, size and density of the particle system, the physico-chemical properties of the drug and the presence of adjuvants. The rate of drug release is faster when the CS-loaded microspheres are smaller in size, due to the smaller diffusion path length for the drug and the larger contact surface area of the smaller particles with the dissolution medium. On the other hand, release is slower when high-molecular-weight CS is used to prepare the microspheres (Sunil, 2004). Today, nanomedicine is expected to lead to breakthroughs in cancer detection, diagnosis and treatment. Among the breakthroughs in nanomedicine, CS nanoparticles are drug carriers that seemed to have the advantage of slow or controlled drug release, improving drug solubility and stability, increasing efficacy and reducing toxicity. In vitro and in vivo studies have also shown that CS has antitumor effects, opening up good prospects for its application as an antitumor drug and drug carrier (Elgadir, 2015). On the other hand, chemical modification of CS gives the possibility of forming autoaggregates (oligomers) in aqueous media. A charge complex can be produced between the cationically charged autoaggregates and the negatively charged plasmid DNA. The feasibility of self-aggregates makes CS an in vitro delivery vehicle for transfecting genetic material into mammalian cells (Sunil, 2004).

I.3.1.7. **CS/ edible chlorogenic acid nanocapsules for prolonged, bio-targeted nutraceutical efficacy**

Nallamuthu et al (2014) encapsulated CS/chlorogenic acid in nanoparticles using the ionic gelation method. This acid is a compound widely found in fruits and vegetables. In the food industry, the encapsulation technique enhances poorly soluble and bioavailable phytocompounds. In addition, their targeting capacity, slow-release properties and substance stability can be significantly modified. Upon ingestion, nanoparticles prepared in fortified foods adhere to the mucosa of the GIT, which is a prerequisite before transit through the body and transport via the bloodstream to various organs. Such a system could prolong the therapeutic effect of nutraceuticals at their specific target sites. For such entrapment purposes, carbohydrates (such as CS) can be used as carrier materials, depending on the nature of the substances to be encapsulated. CS was used in this case for its non-toxicity, biocompatibility, biodegradability and permeation-enhancing properties. To prepare the nanocapsules, CS was first dissolved in an acetic acid solution (the concentration of acetic acid in aqueous solution was 1.75 times that of CS). Under magnetic stirring at room temperature, an aqueous solution of chlorogenic acid (TPP) was added to CS solutions using a peristaltic HPLC pump with a flow rate of 0.2 ml/ min. Finally, we obtained nanoparticle suspensions, where the nanoparticles were separated by centrifugation, then lyophilized and stored at 4°C until further use (in food processing). The evolution of the size and zeta potential (the charge that develops at the interface between a solid surface and its liquid medium) of nanoparticles during heat treatment at 80, 100 and 120°C was studied. There was a rapid reduction in the size and zeta potential of the nanoparticles, during the first 5 minutes of heating, at all temperatures, then later up to 15 minutes, the effect was minimal with a progressive reduction in size and zeta potential. Heat treatment may have affected the adsorption of chlorogenic acid to the surface, as well as the cross-linking structure involved in layer formation. As a result, particle size was reduced and the positive charge on the surface was also altered, which in turn could have caused a decrease in zeta potential. This mechanism takes place relatively quickly as the temperature rises. With further heat treatment, however, particle size and zeta potential were maintained within a regular range, probably because the matrix structure in which chlorogenic acid and CS were combined by ionic gelation inside the particles was more stable than the particle surface. The effect of heat on the nanoparticles was similar to the previous report by Jang et al. for encapsulated vitamin-C. The CS polymer showed a melting point peak at 191.6°C, in acetic acid solution, and the encapsulated nanoparticles did so at 200°C. A slight shift in melting point may be due to the interaction of CS with chlorogenic acid. Since the shift is not too great, we can assume that the encapsulation process has not affected the structure and properties of the CS polymer. In addition, the stability of the nanoparticles at room temperature was studied for one month during storage. They were found to be almost stable in terms of particle size as well as particle zeta potential, indicating the overall stability of the nanoparticles in an aqueous environment at STP. In ionotropic titration, a point is reached where the positive charge is completely neutralized by a negative charge. This point is known as the isoelectric point (Pi), which is defined as the pH at which the net charge of the particle is zero, and is very important from a practical point of view. Pi of nanoparticles was found to be at pH 7.66 indicating the highest stability of these nanoparticles (Nallamuthu, 2014).

I.3.1.8. **CS/silver nitrate antiseptic hydrogels**

Kozicki et al (2016) studied the behavior of CS and silver nitrate hydrogels prepared at 23°C, notably without stirring, and kept in the dark to allow the reagents to interact. CS was dissolved in 1% acetic acid, with several decoctions of concentrations (1; 2; 3; 4 and 5%), before mixing with aqueous silver nitrate (2.5; 5; 7.5 and 10%). Hydrogels were examined by swelling studies in distilled water. After a given time, when the equilibrium swelling point was reached, the samples were dried at 40°C and used against two pathogens Escherichia coli and Bacillus subtilis. All hydrogels consisting of irradiated CS and silver nitrate were effective against both bacterial strains. Because CS solutions in acetic acid, made from non-irradiated CS, revealed no action against them. Whereas powdered solutions of CS absorbing 25; 60; 120 and 200 kGy of gamma radiation revealed antibacterial activity against both bacteria, and no bacterial growth was observed after deposition of even a drop of 2% irradiated CS solution (in 1% acetic acid) on an agar gel containing a bacterial strain. While, it was also found that the dried state of the hydrogels (resembling thin sheets) did not improve their antimicrobial activity, compared to hydrogels in the swollen state. Moreover, by increasing the temperature and decreasing the pH, not only is the solubility of the CS improved, but also its antibacterial activity. According to Kozicki's results, at neutral pH, there are certain intervals in CS molecular weight values {($\leq$ 29.2 kD) & [72.1; 300] kD}, where its antimicrobial activity decreases when there is a decrease in CS molecular weight. Therefore, a clear relationship between the molecular weight of CS and its antimicrobial efficacy cannot really be established. It has been accepted that in the case of the CS reaction with silver nitrate, the cross-linking agent is silver nitrate interacting with the amino groups of chitosan. The higher the concentration of the crosslinking initiator, the more crosslinking can be achieved. Intramolecular cross-linking is favored over intermolecular cross-linking, so nanogels can be formed (internally cross-linked macromolecular coils). On the other hand, the behavior of hydrogels in water depended on the reaction time and the concentration of the CS solution. However, hydrogels with lower stability proved useful for the functionalization of pharmaceutical textile materials, imparting antimicrobial properties (Kozicki, 2016).

1.3.1.9. **Antibacterial edible films with acetic acid/ CS on shredded black radishes**

Edible coatings based on CS and acetic acid could be a good alternative for the inactivation of two different strains of Listeria monocytogenes on shredded black radish. Medium molecular weight CS (Mw: 190-310 kD, DD: 75-85%, Sigma - Aldrich, Germany) was dissolved in a 1% (v/v) acetic acid solution, which was stirred for 24 h to ensure total solubility. The final concentration of CS in the solution was 0.5 and 1% (w/v). Coatings were applied to shredded black radish samples using the same procedure: 10 ml of CS solution was added to 100 g of vegetables. Samples were thoroughly mixed in a biological safety cabinet, then inoculated with 1 ml of bacterial suspension to reach a final concentration of around 104 CFU/ g. All samples were stored in sterile glass jars at 4°C until analysis, which was carried out every 24 h for 7 days. The highest inhibitory activity was observed in coatings prepared with acetic acid and 1% CS. Experimental data indicated that the bacterial strains tested decreased to undetectable levels in black radish samples from the first day of storage until the end of the test (Jovanovic, 2016).

1.3.1.10. **Morphogenic deproteinized bovine bone microsphere scaffolds/ CS**

Bone morphogenic protein (BMP-2) / CS microspheres were successively loaded onto a deproteinized bovine bone (DBB) scaffold. BMP-2 underwent an initial burst release followed by a sustained release. Encapsulated bone morphogenetic protein-2 possessed biological activity. Biocompatibility was good. The microsphere scaffold system may find applications in tissue engineering (Cheung, 2015). CS microspheres loaded with BMP-2 were fabricated by cross-linking. Briefly, CS with a viscosity of 150-900 cP and deacetylation of 75-85% was refined twice by dissolution in aqueous acetic acid solution and precipitation from dilute ammonia. A CS solution (10 g/l) was prepared by dissolving CS in a 2.3% (v/v) aqueous acetic acid solution. 500 mg of this CS solution and the different BMP- 2 contents (0.75 µg/ ml, 1 µg/ ml, 1.25 µg/ ml) were mixed, then the crosslinker was added (vanillin 1% v/ v in an aqueous ethanol solution). The emulsified solution was immediately poured into the CS-BMP-2 mixture and stirred with a magnetic stirrer for 4 h to allow the solvent to evaporate. The hardened microspheres were then collected by centrifugation at 3000 rpm for 3 min, washed three times with distilled water and lyophilized using a freeze-dryer. The preparation of BMP-2-loaded CS microspheres on DBB scaffold surfaces was carried out according to the following process: In the first step, DBB powders were discharged by radiofrequency (RF) plasma in an oxygen-filled chamber at a pressure of 200 mTorr Pa. Plasma power density and treatment time were set at 30 W and 120 s, respectively. Next, the treated DBB powders were mixed with different contents of CS microsphere solution and poured into a polystyrene mold, and frozen at -20°C overnight. Finally, the composites were freeze-dried with a freeze-dryer to obtain the DBB / CS microsphere scaffolds (Li, 2015).

I.3.2. **The theoretical reaction mechanism**

Knowing that the electronegativities of H, C, N and O are 2.2; 2.55; 3.04; and 3.44, respectively (Lide, 2009), and from the data of several previous researches in this chapter (*), we can deduce the following theory:

I.3.2.1. **Step 1:** Although pi bonds are weaker than sigma bonds, a double bond, which consists of a sigma and pi bond, is stronger than a single bond, because there are two bonds, which is why the oxygen of the hydroxyl function in the acetic acid molecule tends more to gain a negative charge than the oxygen of the saturated carbon oxide function in the acetic acid molecule (Ouellette, 2015). Thus, the oxygen of the hydroxyl group in the acetic acid molecule attracts the bond existing between it and the adjacent proton, thereby releasing a hydrogen into the aqueous medium. Then, the free electron doublet of the primary amino groups of the CS in the deacetylated unit attracts the free hydrogen resulting from the acid hydrolysis of acetic acid (*; Lide et al., 2009).

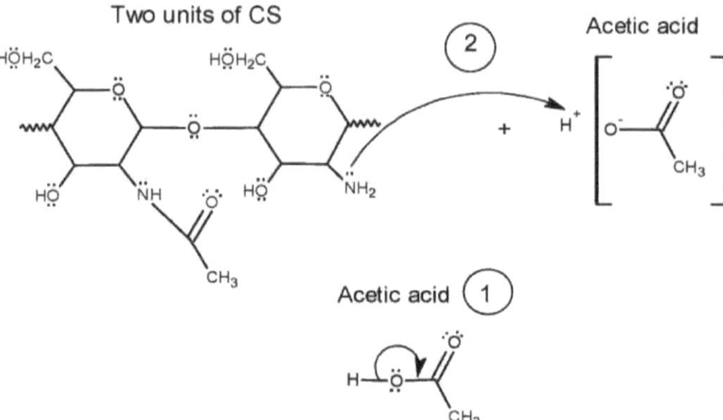

Figure 2. Schematic presentation of stage 1 (the most common).

I.3.2.2. **Step 2:** The nitrogen of the protonated primary amino group attracts a free acetylate anion via its positive charge (*; Lide et al., 2009). A primary ammonium salt of CS is formed. Secondary CS salts are not formed at 1% acetic acid, as this is a weak acid, and the CS amino functions are weak bases (*).

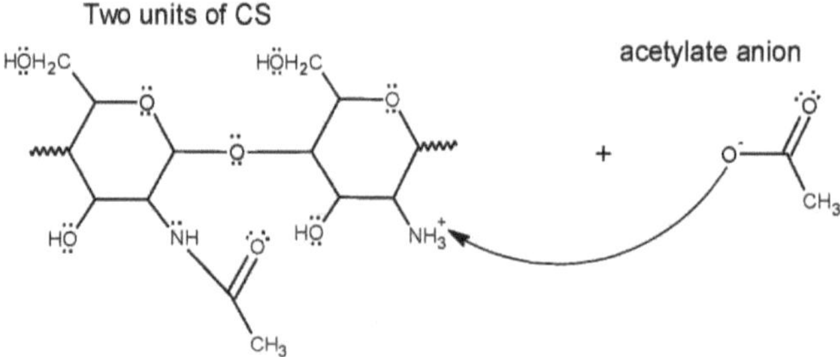

Figure 3. Schematic presentation of step 2.

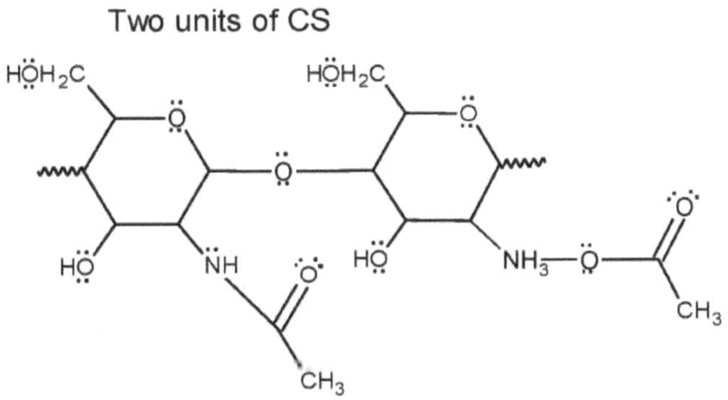

Figure 4. Schematic presentation of step 2 (CS primary ammonium salt).

I.3.2.3. **Stage 3:** The reaction between an acid and an alcohol function is catalyzed by the acid. The acid's hydroxyl function detaches from the acid and bonds with the alcohol's hydrogen, releasing a molecule of water into the medium (Solomons, 2000).

Thus, the oxygen of the methanol function in CS attracts the electron doublet linking it to hydrogen, while the oxygen of the hydroxyl group in acetic acid molecules attracts the electron doublet linking it to the carbon of the carbonyl function (*; Lide et al., 2009).

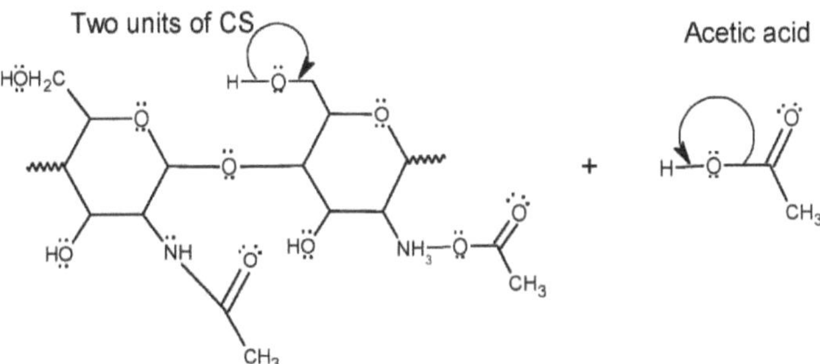

Figure 5. Schematic presentation of step 3.

I.3.2.4. **Step 4:** The oxygen anion formed in the methanol function of CS attracts the carbocation formed after removal of the hydroxyl function from acetic acid, while the removed hydroxyl function attracts free hydrogen from the ethanol function of CS (*; Lide et al., 2009; Solomons et al., 2000).

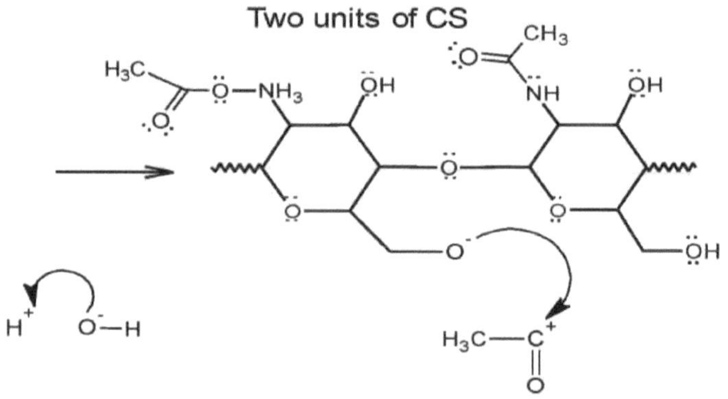

Figure 6. Schematic presentation of step 4.

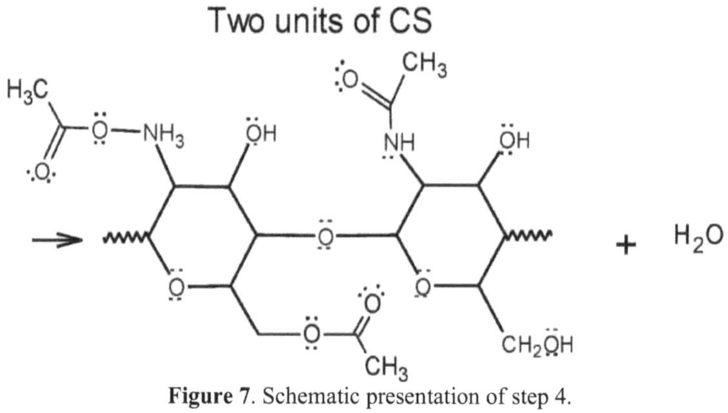

Figure 7. Schematic presentation of step 4.

I.3.2.5. **Step 5:** The oxygen of the primary hydroxyl function in CS attracts the electron doublet linking it to hydrogen, while the oxygen of the hydroxyl group in the acetic acid molecule attracts the electron doublet linking it to the carbon of the carbonyl function (*; Lide et al., 2009; Solomons et al., 2000).

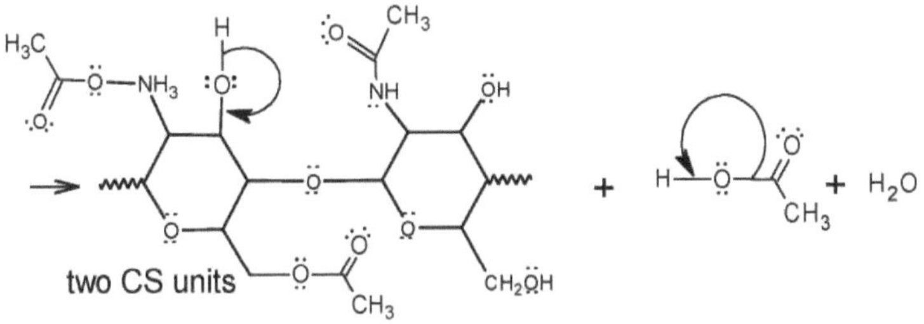

Figure 8. Schematic presentation of step 5.

I.3.2.6. **Step 6:** The oxygen anion formed in the primary hydroxyl function of CS, attracts the carbocation formed after removal of the hydroxyl function from acetic acid, while the hydroxyl function removed from the acid attracts free hydrogen from the methanol function of CS, so a molecule of water is released back into the medium (*; Lide et al., 2009; Solomons et al., 2000).

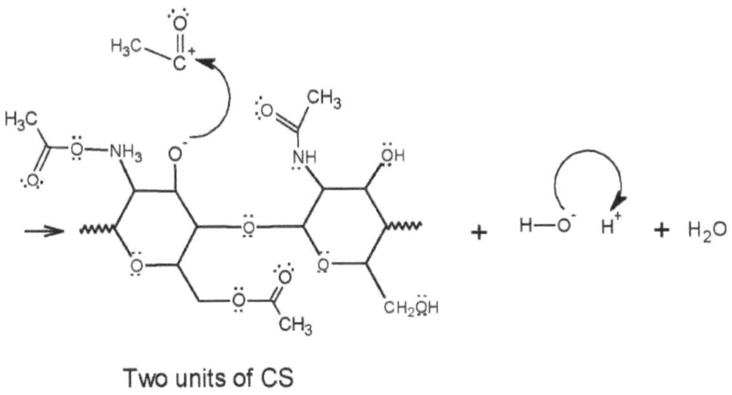

Figure 9. Schematic presentation of step 6.

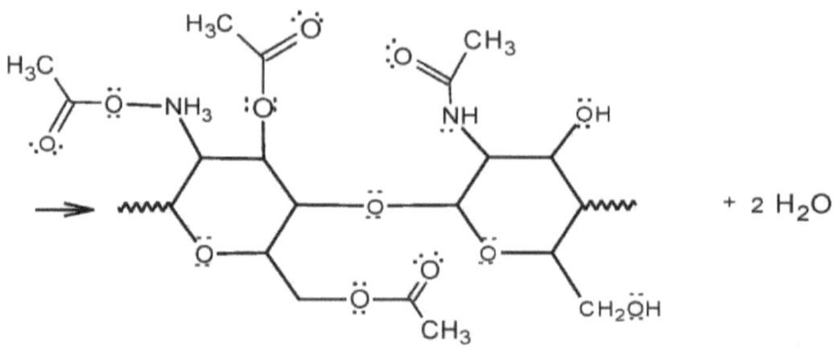

Figure 10. Schematic representation of the final structure when the solubility and isoelectric point of the two CS units, are reached: when CS is dissolved in a 1% aqueous acetic acid solution, at ambient temperature and pressure, pH <6 (*), with continuous (Elsabee et al., 2013; Elgadir et al., 2015) and vigorous (Jawaid et al., 2016; Stiufiuc et al., 2013), and with slow incorporation of CS powder into the solution (Seiller, 1996) and then allowing the suspension to stand still before use (Chiou et al., 2004; Zain et al., 2014; Huang et al., 2004) (Best conditions to stimulate CS nanoparticle formation).

Conclusion Chapter 3

The reaction mechanism presented shows that when the solubility of CS in the aqueous acetic acid solution is reached, under these selected experimental conditions, a primary CS salt is formed between its protonated primary amino groups and the acetylate anions generated by acid hydrolysis of acetic acid: the deacetylated monomer may have up to three positive charges, often the protonated primary amine functions, and less frequently the carbo-cations formed by esterification of the primary or secondary hydroxyl functions to CS. The acetylated monomer of CS could have only two positive charges, under our chosen experimental conditions, the two carbo-cations of the primary and secondary hydroxyl functions of CS. Only the amide bonds (covalent bonds) and a significant number of primary and secondary hydroxyl functions of CS remain in place, after dissolution. Under the effect of purely electrostatic interactions between the various atoms making up the CS chain and the aqueous acetic acid solution (laws of electronegativity), all these cations formed in the CS chain as a result of its dissolution, bind with relative speed to the free acetylate anions present in the solution, depending on their degree of electronegativity, on the distribution of hydrophobic methyl functions constituting the acetamide functions of the CS, and on the ionic concentration in the reaction medium, until the CS reaches an overall neutral charge, and remains in equilibrium with the indissociable mass of CS and the free ions in the medium. When the CS reaches an overall neutral charge, this is known as the polymer isoelectric point, at which point the solubility of the CS is reached. When another anionic molecule, more electronegative than the acetylate anions, is added to this dissolved CS, they easily take their place in the polymer chain, providing a raw material (CS), which is potentially used as an adsorbent for anionic dyes, metal ions, proteins and others.

CS, dissolved in an aqueous acetic acid solution, has a number of industrial applications, and is in particular a gelling stimulator of choice over hydrochloric acid, due to its low capacity to disintegrate hydrogels. This enables the preparation of hydrogels with higher stability. Increasing temperature decreases CS particle size until a stable value is reached, and the smaller the CS nanoparticle size, the more prolonged the drug release.

Under continuous vigorous stirring, with slow incorporation of unirradiated CS powder into an acetic acid solution, and after allowing the suspension to stand, CS nanoparticles should be obtained. Freeze-drying the dilute CS-acetic acid solution yields CS films. Hydrogenation of acetic acid-CS solutions with sodium hydroxide provides a cost-effective method of solubilizing CS, compared with direct solubilization of CS powder. It is important to note that concentrated acetic acid solutions at high temperatures can cause depolymerization of CS. This latter phenomenon will be studied in the future.

References

Bleam, W. (2017). Chapter 6 - Acid-Base Chemistry. In Soil and Environmental Chemistry (Second Edition), 253-331.

Cheung, R.C., TB, N.G., Wong, J.H., Chan, W.Y. (2015). Chitosan: An Update on Potential Biomedical and Pharmaceutical Applications. Marine Drugs. 13, 5156-5186.

Chiou, M.S., Ho, P.Y., Li, H.Y. (2004). Adsorption of anionic dyes in acid solutions using chemically cross-linked chitosan beads. Dyes and pigments, 60, 69-84.

Clegg, S.L., Brimblecombe, P. (1986). The dissociation constant and henry's law constant of HCl in aqueous solution. Atmospheric Environment, 20, 2483-2485.

Daoudi, S. (2010). Synthesis and biological activity of quaternary ammonium salts derived from some alcohols. Magister thesis in Industrial Chemistry, Université USTMB d'Oran, Oran, Algeria, p.20.

Demarger-Andre, S., Domard, A. (1994). Chitosan carboxylic acid salts in solution and in the solid state. Carbohydrate Polymers, 23, 211-219.

Dongre. R. (2018). Chitin-Chitosan: Myriad Functionalities in Science and Technology. IntechOpen Publishers. Isbn: 978-1-78923-407-7.

Elgadir, M.A., Uddin, M.S., Ferdosh, S., Adam, A., Chowdhury, A.J.K., Sarker,

M.Z.I. (2015). Impact of chitosan composites and chitosan nanoparticle composites on various drug delivery systems: A review. Journal of Food & Drug Analysis, 23, 619-629.

Elsabee, M.Z., Abdou, E.S. (2013). Chitosan based edible films and coatings: a review, Materials Science and Engineering, 33, 1819-1841.

Furuike, T., Komoto, D., Hashimoto, H., Tamura, H. (2017). Preparation of chitosan hydrogel and its solubility in organic acids. International Journal of Biological Macromolecules, 104, 1620-1625.

Huang, H., Yang, X. (2004). Synthesis of Chitosan-Stabilized Gold Nanoparticles in the AbsenceZPresence of Tripolyphosphate. Biomacromolecules, 5, 2340-2346.

Jawaid, M., Qaiss, A.E.K., Bouhfid, R. (2016). Nanoclay Reinforced Polymer Composites: Nanocomposites and Bionanocomposites. Springer Singapore, DOI: 10.1007/978-981-101953-1.

Jovanovic, G.D., Klaus, A.S., Niksic, M.P. (2016). Antimicrobial activity of chitosan coatings and films against Listeria monocytogenes, 48, 128-136.

Kozicki, M., Kolodziejczyk, M., Szynkowska, M., Pawlaczyk, A., Le'sniewska, E., Matusiak, A., Adamus, A., Karolczaka, A. (2016). Hydrogels made from chitosan and silver nitrate. Carbohydrate Polymers, 140, 74-87.

le Dung, P., Milas, M., Rinaudo, M. & Desbrières, J. (1994). Water soluble derivatives obtained by controlled chemical modifications of chitosan. Carbohydrate Polymers, 24, 209- 214.

Li, Q., Zhou, G., Yu, X., Wang, T., Xi, Y. and Tang, Z. (2015). Porous deproteinized bovine bone scaffold with three-dimensional localized drug delivery system using chitosan microspheres. BioMedical Engineering OnLine, 14:33, DOI 10.1186/s12938-015-0028-2.

Lide, D.R. (2009). In Handbook of Chemistry and Physics. 89th Edition. CRC Press/ Taylor and Francis, p. 9-98.

Liu, L. (2011). A study of nanochitosans and their applications. Publisher: The Hong Kong

Polytechnic University. UMI 3528702.

Makishima, A. (2017). Chapter 7-Life on Mars From the Martian Meteorite? In Origins of the Earth, Moon, and Life. An Interdisciplinary Approach, 139- 162.

Nallamuthu, I., Devi, A., Khanum, F. (2014). Chlorogenic acid loaded chitosan nanoparticles with sustained release property, retained antioxidant activity and enhanced bioavailability. Asian Journal of Pharmaceutical Sciences, 10, 203-211.

Ouellette, R.J., Rawn, J.D. (2015). Introduction to Organic Reaction

Mechanisms, in Organic Chemistry Study Guide. Chap 3.7, p.32.

Pillai, C.K.S., Paul, W., Sharma, C.P. (2009). Chitin and chitosan polymers: Chemistry, solubility and fiber formation. Progress in Polymer Science, 34, 641-678.

Rinaudo, M., Pavlov, G., Desbrières, J. (1999). Influence of acetic acid concentration on the solubilization of chitosan. Polymer, 40,7029-7032.

Rinaudo, M. (2006). Chitin and chitosan: Properties and applications. Progress in Polymer Science, 31, 603-632.

Seiller, M.; Martini, M.C. (1996). Nanoparticle systems for use in topical dosage forms. In Formes pharmaceutiques pour application locale. Tec & Doc, Lavoisier, Paris, France, chap.17, p.449.

Solomons. T.W.G. (2000). 18.7A. Ester synthesis: esterification. In Chimie organique. Cours, exercices corrigés et CD-Rom. Campus Dunod, 7ème edition, p.734.

Stiufiuc, R., Iacovita, C., Lucaciu, C.M., Stiufiuc, G., Dutu, A.G., Braescu, C., Leopold, N. (2013). SERS-active silver colloids prepared by reduction of silver nitrate with short-chain polyethylene glycol. Nanoscale Research Letters, 8:47.

Sunil, A.A., Nadagouda, N.M., Tejraj, M.A. (2004). Recent advances on chitosan-based micro- and nanoparticles in drug delivery (Review). Journal of Controlled Release, 100, 5 -28.

Thakur, V.K., Thakur, M.K. (2015). Eco-friendly Polymer Nanocomposites: Chemistry and Applications. Springer. DOI: 10.1007/978-81-322-2473-0.

Zain, N.M., Stapley, A.G., Shama, G. (2014). Green synthesis of silver and copper nanoparticles using ascorbic acid and chitosan for antimicrobial applications. Carbohydrate Polymers, 112, 195 202.

Experimental part (II)

Chapter 4: Physical method of Galenic Preformulation of Bionanocomposite Antiseptic Hydrogel from Chitosan and Silver Nitrate.

II.4.1. Introduction Chapter 4

Chitosan (CS), a linear biopolymer made up of d-glucosamine and N-acetyl- d-glucosamine units, with the percentage of d-glucosamine units exceeding 50% [1], has two essential characteristics: cationic nature and chelating capacity, and its antimicrobial action is widely known [2]. Ag + ions and Ag nanoparticles (NPs) are thought to be robust, broad-spectrum antibacterial agents, active against a wide variety of pathogenic bacteria [3]. This is why Ag + has been widely used in many antibacterial biomaterials.

Physical hydrogels are held together by molecular entanglements or non-covalent bonds [1]. Various physical hydrogels mainly composed of chitosan (CS) and silver nitrate have recently been manufactured and are increasingly used in biomedicine [3] as they are cheaper and healthier than others [1]. There are simple methods for making CS-Ag hydrogels, such as gradually pouring the AgNO3 solution over the CS solution in the presence of NaOH and subjecting them to magnetic stirring; in this way Sun et al. (2015) obtained the hydrogel in a matter of seconds [3]. Alternatively, CS and AgNO3 can be mixed directly, then poured into a Petri dish and left to hydrogenate with atmospheric ammonia for a day. This second method by Li et al. (2016), resulted in more biocompatible hydrogels with improved mechanical and antibacterial properties [1]. The method of Kozicki et al. (2016) seems to be the one to avoid: pouring the AgNO3 solution on top of the CS solution and letting them interpenetrate at rest, then swelling them, adding distilled water, as a short reaction time (around <4 h) resulted in brittle hydrogels, even when the AgNO3 concentration was high [2]. CS composites loaded with Ag NPs exhibit remarkably strong antimicrobial activity against Gram-negative or Gram-positive bacteria. However, Ag NPs have high surface energies and tend to aggregate and fuse, leading to processing, storage and application difficulties. Encapsulating Ag NPs in matrix systems could provide an effective approach to preventing aggregation. Droplet microfluidics is an emerging technology for precisely controlling and manipulating fluids to generate monodisperse, uniform micro-sized droplets (Ag NPs loading CS particles (microspheres) allow them to be called CS bionanocomposites) [5] [4]. However, the fabrication of microfluidic devices for droplet formation, handling and applications is generally complicated and costly [6].

The size of Ag NPs can be decreased either by decreasing the AgNO3 concentration or by increasing the CS concentration [7], and one study found that increasing the NaOH concentration had no effect on the size of Ag NPs [4], but this has not been confirmed by other researchers [8-9]. On the other hand, CS particle size can be reduced by decreasing the concentration of CS [4] and increasing the concentrations of AgNO3 [2] and NaOH [4]. Initially, we thought that by playing with the concentrations of the three solutions, we could obtain a physical and antiseptic CS - NPs Ag bionanocomposite hydrogel, but to our surprise the results were negative and contradictory to those found by Sun et al. (2015) [3]. We used the magnetic stirrer and ultrasonic bath for reagent mixing and visual and tactile sensory imaging and analysis to describe some of the physical properties of our products such as color, consistency and thermostability.

II.4.2. Materials and Methods

II.4.2.1. Materials and Chemicals

Chitosan (from crab shell DD ≥ 75%, Sigma-Aldrich, USA); silver nitrate (PM = 169.87, Biochem Chemopharma, France); sodium hydroxide (PM = 40, Biochem Chemopharma, France); glacial acetic acid (100% purity, Sigma-Aldrich, USA); magnetic mixer (100-900 rpm, Stuart, UK); ultrasonic bath (20/80 kHz, adjustable temperature, Elmasonic P, Germany); a manual, adjustable single-channel pipette (1000 to 5000 µL) was used in the study.

II.4.2.2. Preparation of CS - NPs Ag Bionanocomposite Hydrogels with NaOH

Overall, we prepared four different mixtures with a brief introduction of the NaOH solution to the CS - AgNO3 solution. CS - NPs Ag - NaOH bionanocomposites were prepared, using Erlenmeyer flasks, in mixtures 1, 2 and 4 and a cylindrical glass jar in mixture 3, under magnetic stirring (300 rpm at room temperature (21°C on average)), in mixtures 1, 2 and 3 and under ultrasonic vibrations (20 kHz at 30°C) in mixture 4. All samples were stored at room temperature in transparent, sealed containers for observation of their physical properties:

Mixture 1: 100 ml of 1.5% CS in 1% acetic acid (v/v) were mixed with 20 ml of 3% AgNO3 and 10 ml of 1% NaOH for 1 h (at 300 rpm).

Mixture 2: 100 ml 0.1% CS in 1% (v/v) acetic acid was mixed with 20 ml 3% AgNO3 for 2 h (at 300 rpm), then 10 ml 10% NaOH was added and mixing continued, for 1 h (at 300 rpm).

Mixture 3: 100 ml of 1% CS in 1% acetic acid (v/v) was mixed with 5 ml of 10% AgNO3 for 1 h (at 300 rpm), then 10 ml of 10% NaOH was added and mixing continued, for 5 min.

Mixture 4: 100 ml of 0.4% CS in 2% acetic acid (v/v) was mixed with 6 ml of 3% AgNO3 for 1 h (at 300 rpm). The suspension was allowed to stand for 48 h, then divided into four 100 ml Erlenmeyer flasks (25 ml each), and 15 ml 5% NaOH was added to each Erlenmeyer flask. The Erlenmeyer flasks were placed in an ultrasonic bath at 20 kHz and 30°C, for 10-15-30 and 60 minutes respectively.

II.4.2.3. **Preparation of the AgNO3 - NaOH solution**

Manually, qualitative quantities of 5% NaOH and 3% AgNO3 solutions were mixed in a 50 ml beaker.

II.4.2.4. **Preparation of NaOH-free CS - Ag NPs Bionanocomposite Hydrogels**

Overall, we prepared two different samples of CS - NPs Ag bionanocomposite hydrogels, without NaOH. The first sample in a large transparent container, without any addition of distilled water, after the elapsed reaction time of CS with AgNO3 and the second in a small one, with the addition of distilled water after the elapsed reaction time CS / AgNO3 :

Sample 1: In a large transparent glass vial (to widen the field of visual observation), we poured 10 ml of 10% AgNO3 on top of 10 ml of 2% CS solution (in 1% acetic acid). We let the reagents stand and hydrogenate in the sealed container at room temperature, in a bench drawer for 9 months.

Sample 2: In a 50-ml beaker, we poured 10 ml of 10% AgNO3 (mixed 1 h at 100 rpm) onto 10 ml of 2% CS dissolved in 1% (v/v) acetic acid (mixed 24 h at 300 rpm), left the mixture for 7 days at room temperature (21°C on average) after covering the beaker several times with transparent cling film (to increase the opacity of the container). After 7 days of reaction time, we tipped the beaker into a sink and discarded the immersing silver nitrate, then added 22.5 ml of distilled water, to the hydrogel, which we left to stand for 24 h to wash and swell the hydrogel, then discarded the water by tilting the beaker into a sink (results for sample 2 are shown in Appendix A).

II.4.3. Results and discussion

II.4.3.1. Results for Bionanocomposites CS - NPs Ag in the presence of NaOH

The results of the CS - NPs Ag - NaOH bionanocomposites are shown in figures (1114). Mixture 1 produced a yellowish liquid solution (Fig. 11), while mixture 2 (Fig. 12) produced a transparent solution with precipitation of reconstituted CS (brown fibers). The color of blend 1 changed from yellow to black after 9 days under light. The reconstituted CS fibers were brown just after agitation was stopped in mixture 2 and even after two days in the dark, as after two days under light the mixture 2 fibers turned black. Mixture 3 (Fig.13) produced a hydrogel as soon as the NaOH was added: the beige and grayish (inhomogeneous) hydrogel mass rapidly became rigid and highly elastic, and the magnetic rod turned with difficulty, even when the stirring speed was increased, a little gray liquid remained, in excess.

The hydrogel formed in mixture 3 disintegrated after 48 hours, resulting in a small brown mass, floating in a lot of clear liquid, which resembled a small boiled lettuce leaf in its consistency, and disintegration did not progress, within two days. For mixture 4, hydrogenation was locally instantaneous as soon as NaOH was added to the CS - AgNO3 solution, but as the ultrasonic stirring time increased, the amount of transparent liquid increased and the amount of brown hydrogel decreased (Fig. 14). After 24 h, there was the same amount of clear liquid and brown hydrogel mass in all Erlenmeyer flasks, and most of the hydrogel had disintegrated.

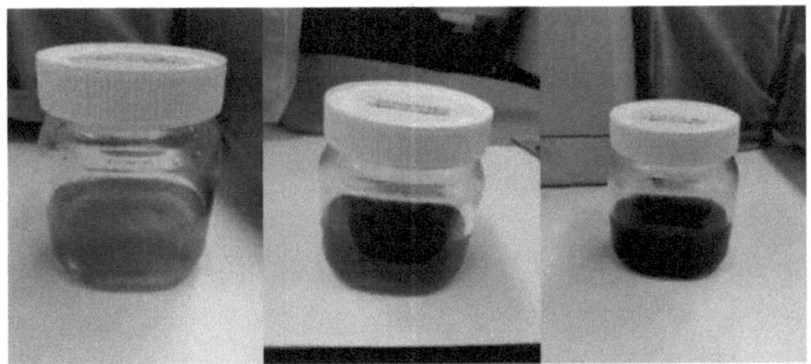

Figure 11. Mixture 1 just after stopping mixing, after 5 days and after 9 days in the light from left to right respectively.

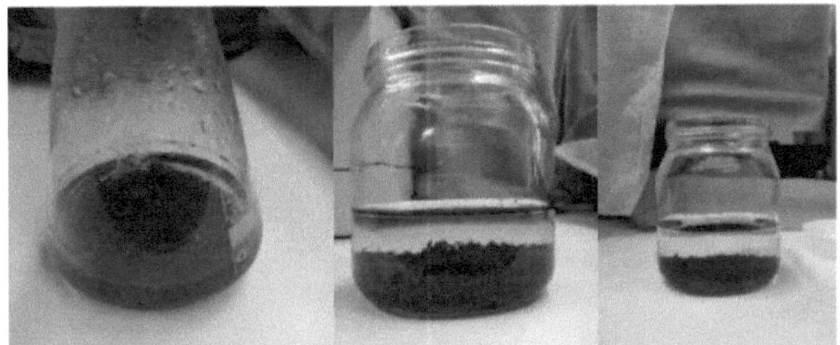

Figure 12. Mixture 2 just after stopping mixing, after 2 days in the dark and then after 2 days in the light from left to right respectively.

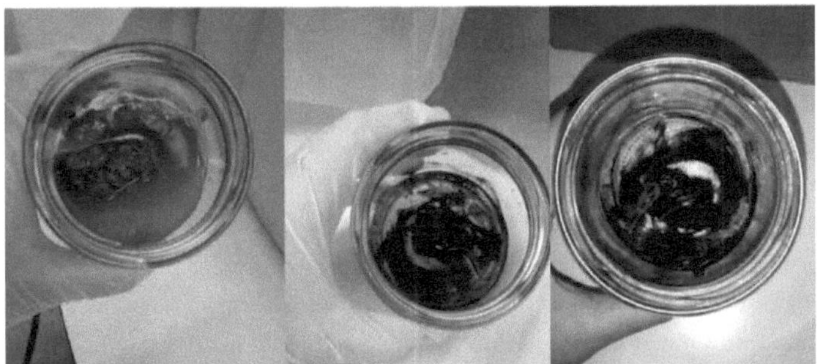

Figure 13. Mixture 3 just after stopping mixing, after 2 days and after 4 days in the dark from left to right respectively.

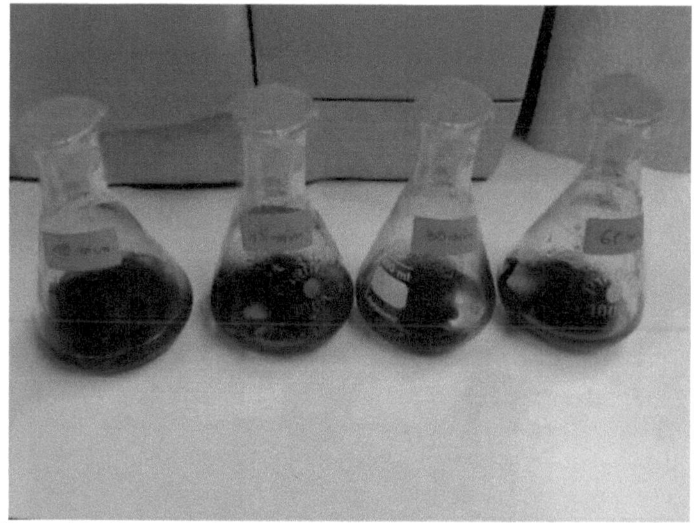

Figure 14. Mixture 4 after 10 - 15 - 30 and 60 min at 20 kHz and 30°C from left to right respectively, just after sonication was stopped.

In summary, we obtained three phenomena when mixing solutions of CS, AgNO3 and NaOH, with mixtures 3 and 4 exhibiting the same phenomena: When the mixing time of the CS solution is long (24h), and if the CS solution is left to stand at 1°C for 5 months before use, and despite the high CS concentration (1.5%), a yellow liquid solution is obtained when the volume fractions of silver nitrate and sodium hydroxide are somewhat high (20 and 10 ml respectively) and their concentrations are low (3% and 1% respectively). With the same volume fractions of the three solutions, but with a shorter mixing time of the CS solution (1h), a lower concentration of CS (0.1%), and a higher concentration of NaOH (10%), keeping the same concentration of AgNO3 (3%), there will be precipitation of the reconstituted CS fibers (brown color) and the solution will remain transparent. By decreasing the volume fractions of silver nitrate and NaOH (5 and 10 ml respectively), while increasing their concentrations (10% for both), and that of CS (1% for 1 h of agitation), there will be instantaneous and heterogeneous hydrogenation (beige and grayish-brown), as soon as NaOH is added, under magnetic agitation. With lower concentrations of CS, AgNO3 and NaOH (0.4% (stirred for 2 h); 3% (stirred for

30 min) and 5% (stirred for 30 min) respectively), and a higher volume fraction of NaOH (projectively 60 ml), keeping those of CS and AgNO3 approximately the same (100 ml and 6 ml respectively), a brittle, heterogeneous brown hydrogel can be instantly obtained, but highly thermosensitive under sonication. In all cases, the hydrogenated proportion disintegrates easily and rapidly (after 24 to 48 h), leaving a brown gummy mass floating in the solution.

II.4.3.2. **Results for the AgNO3 - NaOH mixture**

The results of mixing AgNO3 - NaOH are shown in Figure 5. By mixing a little 5% NaOH solution with a little 3% AgNO3 solution, a cloudy grayish-brown solution was instantly obtained. This explains the appearance of a brown elastic mass in mixture 1, a brownish-gray color in mixtures 2 and 3, and the brown color in mixture 4 as soon as NaOH was added to the CS-AgNO3 solution.

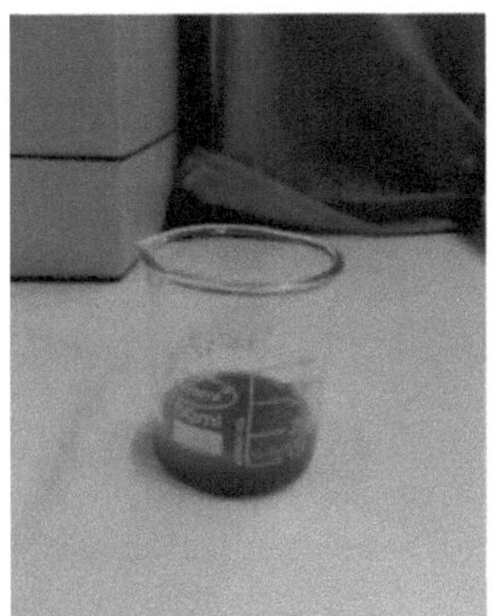

Figure 15. AgNO3 - NaOH solution.

II.4.3.3. **Hydrogel CS - AgNO3 results without NaOH**

The results for the CS-AgNO3 hydrogel, without NaOH, are shown in Figure 16. After 9 months of reaction time, the Ag NPs aggregates clearly appeared, thanks to the instantly formed hydrogel, made of CS and silver nitrate only, which had a very high rigidity, at the end (all the AgNO3 solution was adsorbed by the CS matrix, contrary to what happened in figure (A1 - A2)) and its color changed from transparent to dark brown.

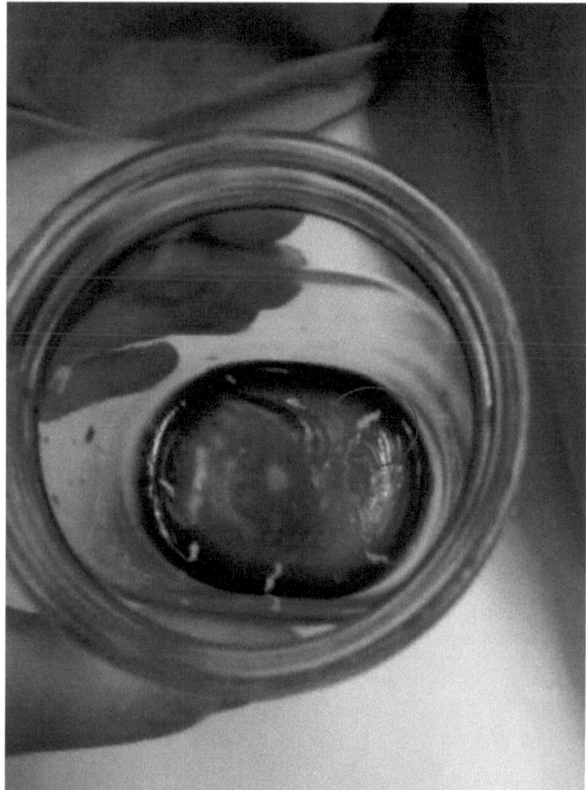

Figure 16. Clear appearance of Ag NPs aggregates (circled in red) in hydrogel made from CS and AgNO3 without NaOH (after 9 months reaction time).

II.4.3.4. **Principle of the study**

The preparation of the bionanocomposite hydrogel CS - NPs Ag- NaOH, was based on a study by Sun et al. (2015), which was based on the multistimuli-sensitive cross-linking, of hydrogels, by metal ions and CS. Sun et al. (2015), mixed the biopolymer CS, with a variety of metal ions, at the appropriate pH values, and they obtained a series of transparent and stable hydrogels (thermal stability for 6 months at room temperature), in a few seconds, by supramolecular complexation. In their study, Sun et al (2015) gradually introduced the 0.3 M silver nitrate solution, into a beaker, containing the 0.4 to 4% wt CS solutions, which were subjected to magnetic mixing. The CS solution was prepared by dissolving in acetic acid (1%), a lower pH value not leading to hydrogenation. The procedure of Sun et al. (2015) was relatively simple, although the hydrogenation time, depended on the concentration of the CS solution. Keeping the same AgNO3 concentration (0.3 M), the higher the CS concentration, the more hydrogenation was delayed.

Curiously, rapid hydrogenation was observed, when Sun et al. (2015) increased the pH values of the CS solutions, by adding NaOH solution (0.2 M). Their prepared hydrogels were elastic in nature, and had good thermostability (could withstand 100 ° C). Each hydrogel had a high water content, exhibiting a relatively low critical gelation concentration (CGC) of less than 1% by weight metal-biopolymer system, lower than that of most reported biopolymer-based supramolecular hydrogels. The hydrogels reacted to a variety of external stimuli, were moldable so that objects of persistent shape could be formed, and could be used in antibacterial gel membranes [3]. In general, antibacterial gel membranes could be used in the treatment of oral inflammatory gingivitis [10] as well as in topical dressings [11] or in water treatment [12].

In the present study, we used NaOH as a gas pedal in the preparation of Ag NPs, stabilized in CS, by reduction with NaOH, as it has been reported, that additional -OH groups, generated in solution, by sodium hydroxide, improve the rate of chemical reduction of Ag ions, and cleaner Ag NPs can be synthesized in seconds [8-9]. In addition, NaOH helps hydrogenate the bionanocomposite [3-4; 8]. On the other hand, Ag NPs are the fillers (charges or also nuclei) in functionalized CS particles. These fillers, rather than "reinforcing" or "re-enforcing" agents, improve the mechanical properties of the CS bionanocomposite, and can promote controlled drug delivery from it [5]. CS characteristics make it highly attractive for use as a reducing and stabilizing agent, enabling efficient synthesis of Ag NPs (CS prevents NPs from agglomerating without interfering with their activity). Since CS already has antimicrobial properties, it is expected that the interaction of these Ag NPs could result in a synergy of their antiseptic properties for potential biomedical applications [13]. When the CS solution reacts with a silver nitrate solution, complexation occurs between the Ag + ions and the CS chains, through the -OH and -NH2 binding sites, thus effectively reducing hydrogen bonding and destroying the crystalline structure of the CS chains. This complexation is attributed to the coordination of Ag + ions, having empty orbitals, to CS chains, which have many free hydroxyl and amino groups with abundant electron, non-bonding doublets [3].

II.4.3.5. Color origins

The percolation of contaminated water, through sheets of paper, containing Ag NPs is a promising way to provide emergency drinking water. Swensson et al. (2018), demonstrated an improved way, to produce Ag NPs, in sheets of paper, by adding sodium hydroxide to the glucose reductant. The blotting papers were left soaked, in an AgNO3 solution, and after draining, were immersed in an alkaline glucose reducing solution prior to drying. The usual yellow-brown coloration of the leaves appeared at room temperature [9]. When Stiufiuc et al (2013), added drop by drop, a solution of AgNO3 to a solution of polyethylene glycol 200 - NaOH (the latter solution was heated to boiling), under vigorous stirring, the color of the solution, changed significantly, to light yellow suggesting that the chemical reaction had taken place and that the grains were available in the solution [14]. Thus, the colors of our final products (the CS - AgNO3- NaOH bionanocomposites) are in coordination with those reported by Stiufiuc et al. (2013) [14] and Swensson et al. (2018) [9], and they originate mainly, from the reaction between the reagents AgNO3 and NaOH (as shown by the color of the AgNO3 - NaOH solution in Figure 15). Although under light, the color changes from yellow to black on the solution of mixture 1 (Fig. 11), from brown to black on the fibers of mixture 2 (Fig.2), and from transparent to dark brown on the CS - AgNO3 hydrogel (Fig. 16), this is explained by the fact that AgNO3 decomposes into Ag, as AgNO3 is photosensitive, which is why silver nitrate solution is generally stored in brown bottles [15]. Furthermore, the final color of our CS - AgNO3 hydrogel, without NaOH (shown in figure (A1 - A2)), confirmed the results found by Kozicki et al. (2016) and Li et al. (2016) and showed that supramolecular complexation between CS and AgNO3, is slightly responsible for the brown color of the hydrogel in the presence of NaOH [1-2].

II.4.3.6. Mixture 1

CS is highly sensitive to environmental conditions, so air temperature can affect the rate of CS degradation, particularly in liquid and semi-solid products. Storage of CS solution, both at ambient and elevated temperatures, resulted in faster degradation of CS chains, and the rate of hydrolysis was found to follow first-order kinetics. Interestingly, no significant chain hydrolysis was observed in the CS solution, stored at 5°C [16], for 60 days [17]. To preserve the initial properties of the CS-based product, preventing damage to the polymer chain, and for long-term stability, it should be stored at a temperature below 5°C, in a closed container. It was found that the higher the degree of deacetylation (DD) of the CS sample, the slower the rate of acid hydrolysis observed during storage. This phenomenon was explained by the fact that CS with a higher DD has a less porous structure, and therefore a lower water absorption capacity (as CS is hygroscopic in nature), which limits the speed of the degradation process in acidic media [16]. In the study by Nguyen et al (2008), different concentrations of 0.8 M, 0.2 M (close to 1% (v/v)) and 0.1 M acetic acid did not affect the rate of degradation of

CS, over 60 days at 28°C [17]. On the other hand, ascorbic acid added to CS dissolved in acetic acid, was found to induce faster degradation at low polymer concentration [18]. Thus, since the DD of our CS was $\geq$ 75% and the CS concentration in mixture 1 was 1.5% (According to the study by Li et al. (2015), there is a significant increase in the viscosity of CS solutions at concentrations above 1.5% by weight, and this was confirmed in Appendix B) [1], they tended to delay its long-term degradation, and it is very likely that the acetic acid concentration of the CS solution in mixture 1 had no considerable effect on the degradation of the CS solution at 1 ° C for 5 months. Thus, it may be suggested that mixture 1 remained liquid not because the CS solution was degraded or very dilute, but because the volume fractions of AgNO3 and NaOH were large in front of their concentrations [1; 16-18].

11.4.3.7.**Mix 2**

Binias et al (2006) achieved total reconstruction of the original supermolecular structure of chitin when using potassium hydroxide solution as an alkaline medium. Dibutyrylchitin fibers were transformed into regenerated chitin fibers when dilute KOH solutions were applied [19]. Viscous CS solutions can be transformed into fibers in various coagulation solutions such as aqueous solutions of : NaOH, KOH [20], ect; and thus the formation of reconstituted CS fibers in mixture 2 can be explained by the presence of a negligible amount of NaOH in the dilute CS solution [19-20]. For low CS concentrations <0.35% (as mentioned in Appendix B), under stirring for 1 h, the addition of high-molecular-weight NaOH ($\geq$ 40 g / mol), which was stirred for ½ h at 300 rpm, even in small quantities (10 ml / 120 ml CS - AgNO3 solution), tends to regenerate CS fibers, instead of promoting supramolecular complexation.

11.4.3.8. Mix 3

However, the role of NaOH in hydrogenation still remains enigmatic: the addition of NaOH to CS solutions functionalized with antibacterial / antifungal metal fillers, has the effect of stimulating their gelation, whether by magnetic mixing [21] or ionotropic gelation [4]; in another study, CS solutions in acetic acid, hydrogenated by addition of NaOH, optimized the amount of acid needed to dissolve CS, compared with CS powder. In Furuike et al. (2017), the stability of the CS-NaOH hydrogel, was confirmed by the stability of its intrinsic viscosity, when stored at room temperature, for 15 days, in sealed glass, even without pasteurization. During hydrogel preparation, NaOH solution was slowly added to the CS solution, until the pH reached 8.5-9.0. The hydrogel obtained was decanted several times, washed several times using distilled water and a centrifuge, and dialyzed against distilled water, until the external solution was neutralized. After dialysis, the CS hydrogel was centrifuged at 14,000 rpm to remove excess water and finally suspended with a blender to obtain a homogeneous gel [22]. In our case, it seems to us that sodium hydroxide and silver nitrate crystals with a high molecular weight (40 and 169.87 g/ mol respectively), and a relatively short mixing time when dissolved (30 min at 300 rpm), pose a big problem in supramolecular complexation, as does the brief introduction of NaOH into the CS - AgNO3 solution. By making a combinatorial deduction from the results obtained in mixtures 3 and 4, we can deduce the following: at room temperature, with brief introduction of NaOH into the CS-AgNO3 solution, if the concentrations of NaOH and silver nitrate are low (<5 and 10% respectively), and when their volume fractions in the bionanocomposite mixture are high (> 10 and 5 ml respectively / (100 ml CS solution of <1% concentration dissolved in [CH3COOH] > 1% for a stirring time > 1 h)), it would be difficult to achieve stable, transparent and homogeneous hydrogenation, even if the magnetic stirring speed is high ($\geq$ 300 rpm). Although, according to the invention by Chen & Xu et al. (2003), it is clear that the disintegration of a CS - NaOH hydrogel in the general case, could stem from the effect of NaOH in CS deacetylation: The lower the CS degree of deacetylation, the more NaOH tends to disintegrate the hydrogel cross-linking (deacetylation in 2 days, at room temperature, if the ratio of NaOH pellets, to Langostino dry lobster shell, to water is approx. 1: 0.1: 1.5, and in an hour or more, in the 100-150°C range, if the previous ratio is about 1: 0.33: 1) after the deacetylation reaction produced by NaOH on the acetyl groups of CS [23]. For this reason, Sudheesh et al. (2012) [21] and Furuike et al. (2017) [22], used a CS with a DD equal to 85% (DD of at least 78% for Furuike et al. (2017) [22]) [21-23]. According to Rinaudo et al. (1993), 100 ml of 1% CS in 0.4% (v/ V) acetic acid, to which 26.7 ml of 25% NaOH is added, if mixed well at a temperature of 100°C, under a nitrogen atmosphere, even with 0.17 g of NaBH4, an antioxidant against CS degradation, could enable CS deacetylation [24]. Projecting these numerical data onto all our blends, it is clear that NaOH added to the CS-AgNO3 solution, is not like a deacetylating agent for the CS polymer, and that necessarily the increase in NaOH concentration must be limited to avoid polymer degradation and deacetylation, thus avoiding hydrogel disintegration [21 24]. It has been reported that CS membranes between 65 and 80% DD provoked marked inflammatory reactions that subsided over time with film degradation and granulation tissue formation, while membranes made of 94% deacetylated CS showed minimal degradation and mild inflammation [25].

II.4.3.9. **Mixture 4**

In the study by Kozicki et al. (2016) the stiffness of the hydrogels increased when the reaction time between AgNO3 and CS solutions (left to stand at 23°C in a dark room) was increased (as in our CS-AgNO3 hydrogel); and very low concentrations of CS ($\leq$ 1%), enabled them to prepare mechanically weak hydrogels, even when the concentration of the metal crosslinking inducer (silver nitrate) was high, this was due to the low number of crosslinked CS chains. Their hydrogels made of 1% CS with 1% acetic acid and even 10% silver nitrate disintegrated in water immediately after immersion. Furthermore, among the disadvantages of the Kozicki et al. (2016) method is the time it takes to complete hydrogenation, as shown in figure (A1-A2).

All this explains the increase in disintegration in mixture 4, when the time of submission to ultrasonic vibrations is increased, even at low frequency (20 kHz) and moderate temperature (30°C) [2]. In a study of CS sludge degradation: for 1% and 2% solutions of CS in acetic acid at pH $\approx$ 4 (solution close to 1% CH3COOH) [27] and 1 h of agitation, in particular, considerable degradation of the

CS system was observed when the temperature was raised to 50°C. As for the 37°C condition, the variation of the degradation rate over time was barely affected (after 169 h). Martini et al. (2016) suggested the existence of a kind of cut-off temperature value (between 37°C and 50°C), for which the elapsed time (t) begins to have a dramatic effect on the degradation rate, so the temperature threshold (30°C) (significant impact for a short sonication time) is not in coordination with the results of Martini et al. (2016), due to the low concentration of CS and the increase in acetic acid concentration and stirring time in the CS solution of mixture 4 [26]. In another study, where Tween 80 was added to the CS solution (as a surfactant) prior to ionotropic hydrogenation with TPP (sodium tripolyphosphate), the initial size of CS NPs was unaffected despite storage of the chemical bionanocomposite hydrogel at 30°C over 28 days, and this at low CS concentration (0.2% resultant concentration after half an hour's stirring of 2% CS in 1% acetic acid), which is why we speak of weak, non-covalent bonds in our hydrogel [28]. In the study by Forrester et al. (2016), sonication of a silica suspension (in deionized water) for a total duration of around 30 min at 20 kHz and room temperature, then subjected to magnetic stirring, led to highly monodisperse or moderately monodisperse samples, and the D_{50} sizes were 100 nm, 214 nm, 430 nm and 1000 nm [29]. For mixture 4, it is likely that the CS concentration of the initial CS solution (0.4% in 2% CH_3COOH for 2 h stirring), the chosen temperature and the sonication frequency induce reversibility of the sol-gel transition of bionanocomposite hydrogels due to the dispersive motion of ions and NPs, or otherwise due to pronounced acid solvation of the polymer [26-29]. It is clear from the literature, however, that nanocrystalline materials can be thermally unstable (i.e. there were NaOH and AgNO3 nanocrystals in mixture 4 that tended to disintegrate the cross-linking through the hydrogel) [30]. By making a combinatorial deduction from the results obtained in mixtures 3 and 4, the following can be deduced: At moderate temperatures, with a brief introduction of NaOH into the CS - $AgNO_3$ solution, if the concentrations of NaOH and silver nitrate are low (<5 and 10% respectively) and when their volume fractions in the bionanocomposite mixture are large (> 10 and 5 ml respectively / (100 ml CS solution of concentration <1% dissolved in [CH_3COOH] > 1% for a stirring time > 1 h)), it would be difficult to achieve stable, transparent and homogeneous hydrogenation, even if the sonication frequency is low or the elapsed time under sonication is high (1 h at 20 kHz and 30 °C).

II.4.3.10. **A few concepts in the preparation of the CS/Ag NPs bionanocomposite hydrogel**

It is important to note from the literature that supramolecular complexation is accompanied by a gain in entropy [31] and also a decrease in the enthalpy of the system [32]. The minimum stirring speed must be well above 100 rpm to form NPs in bionancomposites [33], while slow introduction of NaOH solution into a CS - AgNO3 solution promotes good dispersion of the fillers on the CS matrix, which would be encapsulated by interfacial polymerization [34]. Clearly, the loading efficiency of Ag NPs in the polymer matrix is determined by the time taken to introduce AgNO3 into the reaction medium. A high degree of binding can be achieved by incorporating AgNO3 into CS before adding NaOH, so silver nitrate can be successfully incorporated into the polymer matrix and/or adsorbed onto its surface. However, loading CS with AgNO3 during the particle formation process (when NaOH is added first) results in higher loadings (aggregates of Ag NPs could be formed as in Figure 16) and slower release [3; 35]. Another way of physically gelling CS is the use of в-glycerophosphate combined with temperature (a gel is formed by heating to around 40°C) [36], it provides transparent products that are potentially used as injectable pharmaceutical deposits [31]. Silver nitrate at 0.5% is the standard and most popular silver salt solution used for topical treatment of burn wounds, so Ag NPs from AgNO3 could successfully disinfect hands. However, concentrations in excess of 1% silver nitrate are toxic to tissues (as shown in Figure 16) [30]. On the other hand, an excessive amount of acid is required to dissolve the CS. As a result, the molecular weight of CS decreases considerably as the pH of the solution decreases. The change in the molecular weight of CS in solution is a crucial problem for the use of CS in various fields such as pharmaceuticals, biomaterials and the chemical industry, as it results in a lack of the characteristics of the original CS [26]. Secondly, we need to reduce the mixing time of the CS solution [26; 28] and let it stand for a period ranging from 6 h to one week (as we are not able to check the stability of the CS solution if it is kept for a long time due to dilution in mixture 1) [7; 37-38], as this will improve the viscoelasticity of the CS solution (i.e. to increase the polymer's solubility and facilitate its tendency to cross-link without affecting the solution's viscosity too much (the two-day rest of the CS solution used in mix 4 did not intensify the polymer's acid hydrolysis) [7; 26; 28; 37-38].

Both silver nitrate and NaOH solutions need to be sonicated (even at 20 kHz for

30 min) after magnetic stirring to optimize NPs size and dispersion, if high molecular weight crystals are used in the preparation, or otherwise we need to increase the magnetic stirring time (1 h or more) [29]. The use of nanocrystalline silver nitrate accelerates the release of silver nanoparticles at the hydrogel-skin interface, and gives an immediate antibacterial effect [30]. Ag NPs have shown stronger antibacterial efficacy than zinc oxide and copper oxide NPs and are the most toxic to mammalian cells, making them good antiseptic agents in chitosan hydrogels, which may cause mild side effects such as slight skin irritation at low concentrations [39].

II.4.4 Conclusion Chapter 4

Our results contradict those found by Sun et al. (2015)[3] with regard to the color of the CS -NPs Ag- NaOH hydrogel (not transparent), its stability time, the temperature it can withstand and its homogeneity. Our results and Stiufiuc et al. (2013)[14] show that the supramolecular complexation reaction between CS, AgNO3 and NaOH solutions must be endothermic. Supramolecular complexation is simple and inexpensive, but at the same time Ag NP aggregates could remain present in the reactive medium, at room temperature (temperature, CS and NaOH reagents and stirring speed are not sufficient to disperse them well). Their presence leads to the disintegration of the bionanocomposite, without forgetting that it was also generated by the presence of NaOH, since it is at the origin of the reconstitution of CS fibers in our experiments and in the literature. Supramolecular complexation requiring an increase in the entropy and a decrease in the enthalpy of the system: the famous key factors of Sun et al. (2015)[3] were a higher temperature during stirring (~ up to 40-50 °C) and the slow introduction of NaOH into the CS-AgNO3 solution, and this under vigorous stirring ($\geq$ 300 rpm), then allowing the suspension to rest and hydrogenate at room temperature (preferably $\leq$ 28 °C). To obtain sufficient hydrogel rigidity, we need to optimize the added quantities of AgNO3 and NaOH solutions while increasing their concentrations (as in Mixture 3), we also need to decrease the stirring time of CS Solution (1/2 - 1) h (then let it rest), increase that of AgNO3 and NaOH (we need to sonicate them as well), decrease the concentration of CH3COOH ($\leq$ 1%), slightly increasing that of CS ($\geq$ 1% per 100 ml CS Solution). Once obtained, these Ag CS-NPs bionanocomposite hydrogels could be applied as surgical hand disinfectants, thanks to their supramolecular nature, or otherwise for the healing of superficial topical burns and must be stored at a temperature below 5 ° C to give them a long stability time. However, the phenomena obtained in the presence of NaOH in these bionanocomposites remain manifold, depending on its initial molecular weight, its mixing time during dissolution, and the amount of material in them, as well as the DD of CS.

Acknowledgements: This work was financially supported by the Algerian Ministry of Higher Education and Scientific Research.

Appendix A

According to our experiments, the Ag CS-NPs bionanocomposite hydrogel is easier to obtain by the method of Kozicki et al. (2016) [2] than by the method of Sun et al. (2015)[3] as shown in Figures A1 and A2. Although we note that this considerably reduces the amount of final product.

After 7 days of reaction time, there were two phases, the functionalized CS hydrogel (grayish-brown in color) and the transparent silver nitrate solution submerging it. After 48 h, the hydrogel formed (but its color was less dark than after a week): the progressive adsorption of silver nitrate by the CS matrix had reached the bottom of the beaker (according to the migratory color change). After 24 h of swelling in water, the hydrogel apparently did not swell or lighten in color.

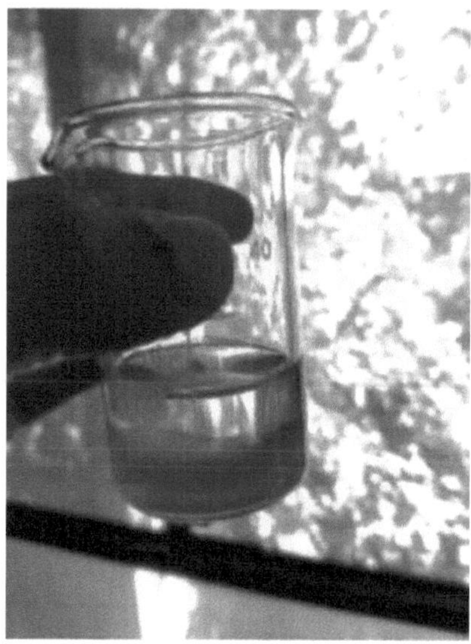

Figure A1. A side view of the CS -NPs Ag bionanocomposite hydrogel without NaOH after 48 h reaction time between AgNO3 and CS solutions (two immiscible phases).

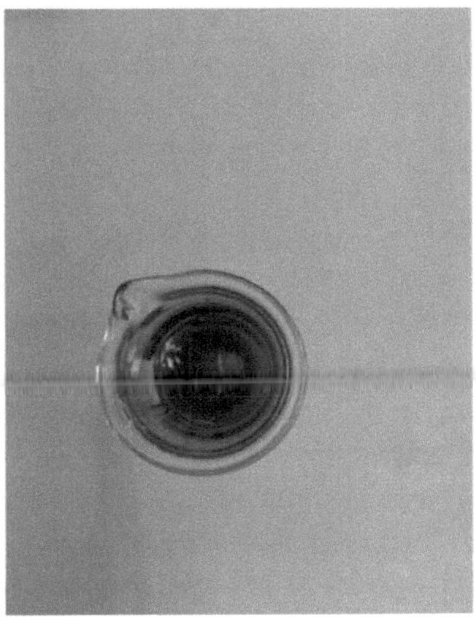

Figure A2. A top view of a small hydrogel sample made from 10 ml of 10% AgNO3 (mixed 1 h at 100 rpm) which was poured onto 10 ml of 2% CS in 1% (v/v) acetic acid (mixed 24 h at 300 rpm), after 7 days resting at room temperature in a highly opaque container, and 24 h swelling in 22.5 ml distilled water.

Appendix B

According to our experiments, the transition of the CS solution (in 1% acetic acid) from dilute to semi-concentrated was observed visually at 0.35% w/v, this result was different from that of Kozicki et al. (2016) [2]. Note that the term "solutions" CS or CS-AgNO3 encompasses colloidal suspensions.

References

[1] . P. Li, J. Zhao, Y. Chen, B. Cheng, Z. Yu, Y. Zhao, X. Yan, Z. Tong, S. Jin. Preparation and characterization of chitosan physical hydrogels with enhanced mechanical and antibacterial properties. Carbohydr. Polym. 157 (2016), 1383-1392.

[2] . M. Kozicki, M. Kolodziejczyk, M. Szynkowska, A. Pawlaczyk, E. Le'sniewska, A. Matusiak, A. Adamus, A. Karolczaka. Hydrogels made from chitosan and silver nitrate. Carbohydr. Polym. 140 (2016) 74-87.

[3] . Z. Sun, F. Lv, L. Cao, L. Liu, Y. Zhang, Z. Lu. Multistimuli-Responsive, Moldable Supramolecular Hydrogels Cross-Linked by Ultrafast Complexation of Metal Ions and Biopolymers. Angew. Chem. Int. Edit. 54 (2015) 7944 -7948.

[4] . L.-S. Wang, C.-Y. Wang, C.-H. Yang, C.-L. Hsieh, S.-Y. Chen, C.-Y. Shen, J.-J. Wang, K.-S. Huang. Synthesis and anti-fungal effect of silver nanoparticles-chitosan composite particles. Int. J. Nanomed. 10 (2015) 2685-2696.

[5] . P.-H. Yassue-Cordeiro, P. Severino, E.-B. Souto, E.L. Gomes, C.-M.-P. Yoshida, M.-A. de Moraes, C.-F. da Silva. Chitosan-based nanocomposites for drug delivery. In Applications of Nanocomposite Materials. Inamuddin; Asiri, A.; Mohammad, A.; USA. 1 (2018) 1-26.

[6] . J.-M. Zhang, J. Qinglei, H. Duan. Three-Dimensional Printed Devices in Droplet Microfluidics. Micromachines. 10(11): (2019) : 754.

[7] . N.-M. Zain, A.-G. Stapley, G. Shama. Green synthesis of silver and copper nanoparticles using ascorbic acid and chitosan for antimicrobial applications. Carbohydr. Polym. 112 (2014) 195-202.

[8] . M. Darroudi, M. Bin Ahmad, A.-H. Abdullah, N.-A. Ibrahim, K. Shameli. Effect of accelerator in green synthesis of silver nanoparticles. Int. J. Mol. Sci. 11 (2010) 3898-3905.

[9] . B. Swensson, M. Ek, D.-G. Gray. In Situ Preparation of Silver Nanoparticles in Paper by Reduction with Alkaline Glucose Solutions. ACS Omega. 3 (2018) 9449-9452.

[10] . C. Benoliel, N. Bertolino, R. Dugue, P. Ferreira-Theret, B. Gutton, L. Haddad, A. Rath- Lavialle, Y. Tillet. Etude de L'Activité Antimicrobienne D'un Gel Buccal: Le Klirich. Laboratoire scientis (2016) 1-18.

[11] . J. Wu, Y. Zheng, X. Wen, Q. Lin, X. Chen, Z. Wu. Silver nanoparticle/ bacterial cellulose gel membranes for antibacterial wound dressing: investigation in vitro and in vivo. Biomed. Mater. 9(3): (2014): 035005.

[12] . J. Zhu, J. Hou, Y. Zhang, M. Tian, T. He, J. Liu, V. Chen. Polymeric antimicrobial membranes enabled by nanomaterials for water treatment. J. Membr. Sci. 550 (2018) 173-197.

[13] . J. Vega-Baudrit, R. Alvarado-Meza, F. Solera-Jiménez. Synthesis of silver nanoparticles using chitosan as a coating agent by sonochemical method. Av. en Quimica. 9 (2014) 125-129.

[14] . R. Stiufiuc, C. Iacovita, C.-M. Lucaciu, G. Stiufiuc, A.-G. Dutu, C. Braescu, N. Leopold. SERS-active silver colloids prepared by reduction of silver nitrate with short-chain polyethylene glycol. Nanoscale Res. Lett (2013) 8:47.

[15] . Q.13, In Competition science vision. Pratiyogita Darpan Group, India (1998) CSV/May/ 1998/443.

[16] . E. Szymanska, K. Winnicka. Review: Stability of Chitosan- A Challenge for Pharmaceutical and Biomedical Applications. Mar. Drugs. 13 (2015) 1819-1846.

[17] . T.-T.-B. Nguyen, S. Hein, C.-H. Ng, W-F. Stevens. Molecular stability of chitosan in acid solutions stored at various conditions. J. Appl. Polym. Sci. 107 (2008) 2588-2593.

[18] . J. Zoldners, T. Kiseleva, I. Kaiminsh. Influence of ascorbic acid on the stability of chitosan solutions. Carbohydr. Polym. 60 (2005) 215-218.

[19] . D. Binias, S. Boryniec, W. Binias, A. Wlochowicz. Alkaline Treatment of Dibutyrylchitin Fibres Spun from Polymer Solution in Ethyl Alcohol. Fibres. Text. East. Eur. 14, (2006) 3 (57).

[20] . L. Notin, C. Viton, J-M. Lucas, A. Domard. Pseudo-dry-spinning of chitosan. Acta Biomater. 2 (2006) 297-311.

[21] . P-T. Sudheesh-Kumar, V. Kumar-Lakshmanan, T.-V. Anilkumar, C. Ramya, P. Reshmi. Flexible and Microporous Chitosan Hydrogel/Nano ZnO Composite Bandages for Wound Dressing: In Vitro and In Vivo Evaluation. ACS Appl. Mater. Interfaces. 4 (2012) 2618-2629.

[22] . T. Furuike, D. Komoto, H. Hashimoto, H. Tamura. Preparation of chitosan hydrogel and its solubility in organic acids. Int. J. Biol. Macromol. 104 (2017) 1620-1625.

[23] . L.-F. Chen, Q. Xu, A.-M. Mueting. Chitosan and methods of producing same. PCT, (2003), WO 03/105590 A1, p.2.

[24] . P. Le Dung, M. Milas, M. Rinaudo & J. Desbrières. Water soluble derivatives obtained by controlled chemical modifications of chitosan. Carbohydr. Polym. 24 (1994) 209- 214.

[25] . Y. Yuan, B.-M. Chesnutt, W.-O. Haggard, J.-D. Bumgardner. Deacetylation of Chitosan: Material Characterization and in vitro Evaluation via Albumin Adsorption and Pre-Osteoblastic Cell Cultures. Materials. 4 (2011) 1399-1416.

[26] . B. Martini, S. Dimida, E. De Benedetto, M. Madaghiele, C. Demitri. Study on the degradation of chitosan slurries. Results Phys. 6 (2016) 728-729.

[27] . C.-K.-S. Pillai, W. Paul, C.-P. Sharma. Chitin and chitosan polymers: Chemistry, solubility and fiber formation. Prog. Polym. Sci. 34 (2009) 641-678.

[28] . W.-R. Handani, W.-B. Sediawan, A. Tawfiequrrahman, Wiratni, Y. Kusumastuti. AIP Conference Proceedings. 1840 (2017) 080001.

[29] . D.-M. Forrester, J. Huang, V.-J. Pinfield. Characterisation of colloidal dispersions using ultrasound spectroscopy and multiple-scattering theory inclusive of shear-wave effects. Chem. Eng. Res. Des. 114 (2016) 69-78.

[30] . B.-S. Atiyeh, M. Costaglioba, S.-N. Hayek, S.-A. Dibo. Effect of silver on burn wound infection control and healing: Review of the literature. Burns. 33 (2007) 139-148.

[31] . J. Nilsen-Nygaard, S.-P. Strand, K.-M. Varum, K.-I. Draget, C.-T. Nordgard. Review: Chitosan: Gels and Interfacial Properties. Polych. 7 (2015) 552-579.

[32] . N.-L. Chekirou. Study of associative processes of β- cyclodextrin inclusion complexes by quantochemical and Raman spectroscopic methods. PhD thesis, University of Oran 2, Oran, Algeria (2012) p.45.

[33] . H. Fessi, J.-P. Devissaguet, C. Thies. Process for the preparation of dispersible colloidal systems of a substance in the form of nanoparticles. French

Invention Patent (1988) PV 86 18446, p.4.

[34] . Seiller, M.; Martini, M-C. Nanoparticle systems for use in topical dosage forms. In Formes pharmaceutiques pour application locale. Tec & Doc, Lavoisier, Paris, France (1996) chap.17, p.449.

[35] . L. Zhaparova. Synthesis of Nanoparticles and Nanocapsules for Controlled Release of the Antitumor Drug Arglabin and Antituberculosis Drugs. Ph.D. Thesis, Technische Universiteit Eindhoven, Eindhoven, The Netherlands (2012) 17-20.

[36] . M. Rinaudo. Chitin and chitosan: Properties and applications. Prog. Polym. Sci. 31 (2006) 603-632.

[37] . Chiou, M.S.; Ho, P.Y.; Li, H.Y. Adsorption of anionic dyes in acid solutions using chemically cross-linked chitosan beads. Dyes Pigments. 60 (2004) 69-84.

[38] . H. Huang, X. Yang. Synthesis of Chitosan-Stabilized Gold Nanoparticles in the Absence/Presence of Tripolyphosphate. Biomacromolecules. 5 (2004) 2340-2346.

[39] . Bondarenko, O.; Juganson, K.; Ivask, A.; Kasemets, K.; Mortimer, M.; Kahru, A.Toxicity of Ag, CuO and ZnO nanoparticles to selected environmentally relevant test organisms and mammalian cells in vitro: a critical review. July 2013, Volume 87, Issue 7, pp 1181-1200.

Chapter 5: Simulations of the Chitosan / Nanosilver Bionanocomposite Hydrogel Manufacturing and Characterization Processes.

II.5.1 Introduction

Chitin is an organic substance (polysaccharide), nitrogenous, flexible and resistant, which makes up the integuments of arthropods (insects and other articulated animals) [1] [2]. Chitosan is obtained after deacetylation of chitin, and is used in the treatment of infections, inflammations and cancers [3].

Silver is a white precious metal, rare in its natural state, but existing in some places in significant quantities, which has facilitated its research and use. The concentration of silver in the litosphere reaches 2.10^{-5} % by weight. Its main derivatives correspond to univalent silver: they are the nitrate AgNO3 and the hydroxide AgOH, which is a strong base. This metal is not oxidized by atmospheric oxygen, but blackens in ordinary air (which contains traces of hydrogen sulfide). It dissolves oxygen when hot and liquid, and during solidification, the oxygen is released, causing the metal to swell, which is how silver solidifies [4].

Silver nitrate is certainly the most important industrial compound of this metal. It is used in the preparation of photographic emulsions. It is highly soluble in water [5]. Silver nitrate, like silver halide, has numerous crystal structure defects, notably due to the fact that the atoms are not all regularly located at the nodes of the crystal lattice, but will settle in interstitial positions with the creation of a hole (Frenkel defect), to a lesser extent, the vacancies are due to both types of atoms (Schottky defect), without interstitial positions appearing. The presence of structural defects is the basis for the use of silver salt emulsions in a gelatin support to make photographic films and plates, for example [4].

In addition to its applications in photography, silver is also used in catalysis. Silver is also used in medicine and dentistry. Its resistance to chemical agents and oxidation, even at high temperatures, means it is used in mechanical engineering, in the manufacture of electrical contactors and in certain high-tech industries (atomic industry). The aerospace industry uses almost as much silver as the photographic industry [5]. In this study, we presented well-founded predictions if we were to carry out in-depth pH and microbiological analyses of these CS / silver nitrate biononanocomposite hydrogels, and at the end, we showed what we would observe if pieces of hydrogel samples were placed on the scanning electron microscope.

II.5.2. Materials and Methods

II.5.2.1. Materials and Chemicals

Chitosan fibers (from crab shells DD $\geq$ 75%, average molecular weight, Sigma-Aldrich, USA); Silver nitrate crystals (MW=169.87, Biochem Chemopharma, France); Sodium hydroxide crystals (MW=40, Biochem Chemopharma, France); Glacial acetic acid solution (100% purity, Sigma-Aldrich, USA); Sodium alginate powder (Sigma-Aldrich, USA) ; Heated magnetic mixer (100-900 rpm, 25-300°C, Stuart, UK); Stable manual micropipettes 100; 500 µL and adjustable micropipette 1000-5000 µL/ pH meter/ SEM-EDX Quanta 250 with tungsten filament (from FEI, USA).

II.5.2.2. Methods

11.5.2.2.1. The different solutions

* **Chitosan suspension (CS):** Slowly incorporate CS into 100 ml aqueous acetic acid 0.3- 0.4- 0.5- 0.6 and 0.7% (v/V), bring to 400 rpm and CSTP for 30 min, then leave to stand for 24 h at room temperature.

* **AgNO3 solution:** In a 200 ml Erlenmeyer flask, dissolve 5 g silver nitrate in 100 ml distilled water and stir at 400 rpm for 1 h.

* **NaOH solution:** In a 200 ml Erlenmeyer flask, dissolve 10 g NaOH in 100 ml distilled water, 400 rpm, 1 h.

* **Surfactant solution (physical gelling agent):** In a 50-ml beaker, dissolve 3 g surfactant (sodium alginate) in 30 ml distilled water and run at 100 rpm for 1 h.

11.5.2.2.2. Nanogel:

On a heated magnetic stirrer, at 400 rpm and room temperature: The entire CS suspension was put in, 10 ml of silver nitrate solution was added. We mixed them for 30 min. Then we adjusted the temperature to 30°C for 10 min, and to

40°C for another 10 min, finally we adjusted the temperature again to 30°C, with stirring at 400 rpm. Next, 10 ml NaOH (1 ml/3 min) was poured in and 4 ml surfactant was added (1 ml/5 min). The mixture was left to stand to hydrogenate for 24 h at room temperature. Then we refrigerated the finished products at T ≤ 5°C for long-term stability.

11.5.2.2.3. Evaluation of Hydrogel pH as a function of Acetic Acid Concentration in CS Suspensions without Surfactant Addition

* **Chitosan suspensions:** Five suspensions of CS at 0.4 (m/V) % were prepared according to parts II.5.2.2.1 and II.5.2.2.2: at 0.3 - 0.4- 0.5- 0.6- 0.7 % (v/V) aqueous acetic acid.

11.5.2.2.4. Evaluation of Hydrogel pH as a Function of Acetic Acid Concentration in CS Suspensions with the Addition of Surfactant

* **Chitosan suspensions:** Five suspensions of CS at 0.4 (m/V) % were prepared according to sections II.5.2.2.1 and II.5.2.2.2: at 0.3 - 0.4- 0.5- 0.6- 0.7 % (v/V), 4 ml of solution of the gelling agent (sodium alginate) were added to each sample.

11.5.2.2.5. Microbiological analysis

The different solutions

* **Chitosan suspensions:** Four solutions of 0.4 (m/V) % CS in 0.3 (v/V) % acetic acid were prepared in accordance with sections II.5.2.2.1 and II.5.2.2.2. * **AgNO3 or NaOH solution**: part II.5.2.2.1. * **ZnO solution:** 5 g were dissolved in 0.5% (v/V) CH3COOH, 400 rpm, 1 h. * **Gelling agent solution:** 4 ml of 10 (m/V)% sodium alginate solution were added to two CS suspensions respectively, as described in parts II.5.2.2.1 and II.5.2.2.2.
I I.5.2.2.2.

* **Nanogels:** we manufactured two highly physical bionanocomposite hydrogels (CS- AgNO3 and CS-ZnO) and two weakly physical bionanocomposite hydrogels with the same antimicrobial agents as described in section II.5.2.2.2.

Microbiological testing of specific microorganisms

Pseudomonas aeruginosa: 100 ml of liquid medium with casein and soybean peptones were seeded with a volume corresponding to 0.1 ml of *P. aeruginosa* storage suspension (gram -) and 1 g of hydrogel was added (1 ml of hydrogel could be added otherwise). The mixture was homogenized and incubated at 37°C for 48 h. 1 ml of liquid from the flask was placed on a Petri dish (9 cm diameter) filled with 15 ml agar-ketrimide medium. The dish was taken up and incubated at 37°C for 48 h. The product passed the test if no microbial growth was observed (pale rods with a greenish-yellow halo).

Staphylococcus aureus: 100 ml of casein and soybean peptone liquid was inoculated with a volume corresponding to 0.1 ml of *S. aureus* (gram+) storage suspension and 1 g of hydrogel was added. The mixture was homogenized and incubated at 37°C for 48 h. 1 ml of the liquid from the vial was placed on a Petri dish (9 cm diameter) filled with 15 ml of Baird Parker agar medium and incubated at 37°C for 48 hrs. The growth of round black Gram-positive colonies surrounded by a clear zone indicates the presence of *S. aureus*. The product passes the test if no microbial growth is detected on Baird-Parker agar.

11.5.2.2.6. **Analysis of Silver Nanoparticles by UV-Visible Spectroscopy**

• **Standard solution:** 100 mg (0.1 g) AgNO3 was dissolved in a 200-ml Erlenmeyer flask and filled with double-distilled water (100 ml), stirred for 1 h at 400 r.p.m.. We took 1 ml of this solution and added 9 ml of bidistilled water, mixing for 5 min. Silver nitrate absorption peaks at 305 nm.

• **Solution Tested:** 200 mg (0.2 g) of hydrogel was dissolved in a 100-mL bottle, filled to the mark with double-distilled water, closed and shaken by hand slowly for a few seconds. 1 ml of the latter solution was taken and 9 ml of bidistilled water was added to a 10 ml bottle, the small bottle was closed and gently shaken by hand.

• **Note:** If there is an absorption band in the UV-visible spectrum that converges towards 420 nm (centered around 420 nm), silver nanoparticles are present.

11.5.2.2.7. **Scanning Electron Microscopy (SEM) analysis**

• **Morphology analysis of CS suspensions:** We prepared a 0.4 (w/V) % CS solution in 0.3 (v/V) % aqueous acetic acid, as described in the operating protocol above (400 r.p.m, CSTP, 30 min, then 24 h rest). We placed the sample under a microscope at a scale of 1000 nm.

• **Morphology analysis of sodium alginate suspensions:** We prepared a sodium alginate solution: in a 50-ml beaker, we dissolved 3 g sodium alginate in 30 ml distilled water and stirred at 100 rpm for 1 hour. We placed the sample under a microscope at a scale of 1000 nm.

• **Morphology analysis of CS / Sodium Alginate suspensions:** We prepared two suspensions of 0.4 (w/V) % CS in 0.3 (v/V) % aqueous acetic acid as described in section 5.2.2.1, and added only 4 ml (1 ml/5 min) of 10 and 15 (w/V) % sodium alginate suspensions respectively, mixing them as described in sections 5.2.2.1 and 5.2.2.2. Both samples were viewed at 1000 nm.

• **Morphology analysis of CS / AgNO3 suspensions:** We prepared a 0.4 (m/V) % CS solution in 0.3 (v/V) % aqueous acetic acid, as described in the operating protocol above (400 r.p.m, CSTP, 30 min, then 24 h rest). We added 10 ml of 5 (w/V)% AgNO3 solution. We mixed them for 30 min with CSTP at 400 rpm. We then adjusted the temperature to 30°C for 10 min, then to 40°C for a further 10 min, at 400 rpm. stirring speed. We saw the sample at 1000 nm.

- **Morphology analysis of CS/ AgNO3/ NaOH suspensions:** We prepared highly physical bionanocomposite hydrogels according to sections 5.2.2.1 and 5.2.2.2, at 0.4% CS in 0.3- 0.4- 0.5- 0.6- 0.7 (v/V) % CH3COOH, 5% AgNO3, 10% NaOH. The samples were viewed at 1000 nm.

- **Morphology analysis of CS/ AgNO3/ NaOH/ Sodium Alginate suspensions:** We prepared weakly physical bionanocomposite hydrogels according to parts 5.2.2.1 and 5.2.2.2, at 0.4% CS in 0.3- 0.4- 0.5- 0.6- 0.7 (v/V) % CH3COOH, 5% AgNO3, 10% NaOH, 10% sodium alginate. Samples were viewed at 1000 nm.

II.5.2.3. **Results and discussion**

II.5.2.3.1. **Apparent pH results for Hydrogel samples**

Table 1: Apparent pH results for several hydrogel samples without sodium alginate are presented in the table below [3] [6].

[CH3COOH] (v/ V) % (v/ V) % (v/ V) % (v/ V) %				
0.3	0.4	0.5	0.6	0.7

(v/ V)					
Apparent pH of hydrogels without gelling agent	9.300	9.363	9.411	9.451	9.484

Table 2: Apparent pH results for several hydrogel samples, with the addition of sodium alginate, are presented in this table below [3] [6] [7] [8].

[CH3COOH] (v/ V) % (v/ V) % (v/ V) % (v/ V)	0.3	0.4	0.5	0.6	0.7
Apparent pH of hydrogels with sodium alginate addition	8.960	9.022	9.071	9.110	9.144

II.5.2.3.2. Results of several Microbiological Analyses of Hydrogel Samples

Whether the hydrogels were highly or weakly physical bionanocomposites based on zinc oxide or silver nitrate, the results were negative, with no bacterial colonies detected [9] [10] [11].

11.5.2.3.3. UV-Visible Analysis Results

According to the various visible UV Spectrograms, the absorption peaks centered around 420 nm for all 10 hydrogel samples, except that peak resolution was improved by increasing the acetic acid concentration in the hydrogel samples of the highly physical bionanocomposite hydrogels, and was also improved by the addition of sodium alginate in the weakly physical bionanocomposite hydrogel [12] [13] [14].

11.5.2.3.4. **Scanning Electron Microscopy results**

• **Results of Morphological Analysis of CS and Sodium Alginate Suspensions**

From the SEM image illustrating the morphology of the CS or sodium alginate polymers, it was clear that the morphology of the CS was not smooth but had a certain roughness. The same was true of sodium alginate.

• **SEM analysis results for CS / Silver Nitrate Mixture**

It should be remembered that AgNO3 was initially in crystalline form. In the figure illustrating the SEM analysis for the CS/AgNO3 mixture, it was not easy to detect the presence of this filler in the CS matrix, since a few holes appeared on the matrix alone, but this does not prevent some changes appearing on the CS morphology after the introduction of this low percentage of AgNO3.

• **SEM analysis results for CS Seul, CS/AgNO3 and CS/AgNO3/NaOH systems**

From the comparison of SEM topographies between CS alone, CS / AgNO3 and CS / AgNO3 / NaOH systems, it became clear that holes and cavities in the CS matrix increase after the addition of each chemical substrate [15], particularly NaOH which is known for its use in CS fiber reconstitution despite its ability to reduce metal crystals such as silver [3].

• **Results of Comparison between Morphology of CS Alone and CS / 10 or 15% Sodium Alginate Systems**

From the SEM images of the 10 and 15% CS / sodium alginate systems, it was very clear that there is a difference between the morphology of pure CS, and those of CS / sodium alginate mixtures with 10 and 15% sodium alginate. It was quite clear that the insertion of a small percentage of sodium alginate into the CS matrix created holes or voids that did not exist in the pure CS matrix. The number of these holes increased as the percentage of sodium alginate in the mixture increased.

- SEM results for CS / sodium alginate and CS / sodium alginate / NaOH / AgNO3 mixtures

A similar comparison was made between SEM images of the CS/sodium alginate and CS/sodium alginate/NaOH/AgNO3 systems: we found that, in the presence of NaOH and AgNO3, the CS/sodium alginate mixtures did not show any holes as in the systems without fillers [15].

II.5.3. Conclusion Chapter 5

The pH results showed that the finished product is weakly basic without rinsing and swelling with distilled water, it is less basic with the addition of sodium alginate, so it needs to be rinsed and swelled several times with distilled water to neutralize it [16].

In conclusion, it was deduced that the presence of AgNO3 and NaOH in CS/sodium alginate matrices has a direct effect on polymer morphology. Moreover, holes appeared in the morphology of CS/sodium alginate blends, compared with pure CS. These holes mean that the addition of a small percentage of sodium alginate to the CS matrix influences its overall morphology, probably reflecting the development of electrostatic interactions between these two oppositely charged matrices during blending. The presence of AgNO3 and NaOH does not necessarily favor the development of such interactions. The charges, also known as bionanocomposite hydrogel reinforcement, insert themselves into the polymer matrices, preventing the appearance of holes, when supramolecular complexation equilibrium is reached [15].

The characterization of dynamic viscosity remains to be reviewed to find the best spreading range on the skin of these topical antiseptic hydrogels, with validated antibacterial properties. A cone-plane rheometer is the best choice for measurement, to optimize the quantity of hydrogel required for analysis, which is generally either a strong or weak rheofluidizing polymer suspension, depending on its consistency [17].

References

1. Dictionnaire HACHETTE, Langue Française, Encyclopédie, Noms Propres, SPADEM- ADAGP Paris, 1980, p. 244.

2. Larousse de la Langue Française, Librairie Larousse, ISBN 2-03-101 301-7, 1977, p. 336.

3. M. GANDI, H. ZEMMOURI, M. AMARI. Research on bionanocomposites of therapeutic value, Booktopia, Science, Non-Fiction, Religion & Beliefs,

Aspects of Religion for NonChristians, Theology , 2021, 60p.

4. La Grande Encyclopédie, Librairie Larousse, ISBN 2-03-000900-8, by SPADEM and ADAGP, 1972, p. 975.

5. Grande Encyclopédie Alpha des Sciences et des Techniques, Chimie, Instituto Geographico de Agostini, Novara, 1973. Grange Batelière, Paris, 1976. Editiond Atlas, Paris, 1976, p.58.

6. H. MEKATEL. Cours et Travaux Dirigés en Electrochimie, Deuxième Année Licence S.T, Système LMD, FGMGP, USTHB, promotion 2013/2014.

7. P. WERLE, J.-P. D'IVENOIS, Livre pharmacie galénique. la concentration en gélifiant, 2ème édition Maloine, 2012, p. 202.

8. N. BALES. PEGs. DESS DE COSMETOLOGIE: *Tableau 4: Utilisation des PEGs en cosmétique,* UQAC, 2014, p. 18.

9. P. Li, J. Zhao, Y. Chen, B. Cheng, Z. Yu, Y. Zhao, X. Yan, Z. Tong, S. Jin. Preparation and characterization of chitosan physical hydrogels with enhanced mechanical and antibacterial properties. Carbohydr. Polym. 157 (2016), 1383-1392.

10. P.-T. Sudheesh-Kumar, V. Kumar-Lakshmanan, T.-V. Anilkumar, C. Ramya, P. Reshmi. Flexible and Microporous Chitosan Hydrogel/Nano ZnO Composite Bandages for Wound Dressing: In Vitro and In Vivo Evaluation. ACS Appl. Mater. Interfaces. 4 (2012) 2618-2629.

11. Microbiological testing of non-sterile products (2.6.13) : Testing for specified microorganisms, European Pharmacopoeia 6.0.

12. M. GANDI. Quality controls of a drug in tablet form: folic acid research/UV dosing of folic acid in a dosage unit. Better World Books, Editions Universitaires Européennes, 2018, 108 p. ISBN-13: 9786202283106.

13. M. Kozicki, M. Kolodziejczyk, M. Szynkowska, A. Pawlaczyk, E. Le'sniewska, A. Matusiak, A. Adamus, A. Karolczaka. Hydrogels made from chitosan and silver nitrate. Carbohydr. Polym. 140 (2016) 74-87.

14. Isabelle Goujon. Alginates, excipients of marine origin used in the pharmaceutical industry: applications to the synthesis of a chemical gel. Pharmaceutical Sciences. 2004. hal-01732836.

15. K. BOURICHA, S. KEDACHI. ELABORATION AND

CHARACTERIZATION OF BINARY SYSTEMS BASED ON BIOPOLYMERS. Master's thesis, FCH, USTHB, 2021, 41 p.

16. T. Furuike, D. Komoto, H. Hashimoto, H. Tamura. Preparation of chitosan hydrogel and its solubility in organic acids. Int. J. Biol. Macromol. 104 (2017) 1620-1625.

17. H. Abchiche. Cours et Travaux Dirigés en Rhéologie des fluides, 1ère Année Master, FGMGP, USTHB, promotion 2015/ 2016.

Chapter 6: Acrylic Acid as a New Generator of Chitosan Bionanocomposite Hydrogels Like Acetic Acid Before.

II.6.1 Introduction

Various studies on hydrogels have been carried out on the polymerization of acrylic acid in the presence of chitosan, generally ammonium persulfate is used as initiator, but the exact mass ratio of initiator to acrylic acid to chitosan in hydrogels, remains hidden in the Literature. These systems have been beneficial for the controlled release of active substances and antibacterial agents, and their mechanical properties have been improved with various processes [1-6]. Acrylic acid seems to be a new generator of chitosan bionanocomposite hydrogels as is acetic acid often used previously [7]. This mini-review is a survey of the various works that have been published on this chitosan/acrylic acid system over the last 5 years [1-6].

II.6.2. Reported work

Bashir et al (2017), have synthesized a novel hydrogel formulation suitable and effective, for drug delivery application. In their study, Bashir et al. were the first to synthesize novel formulations of N-succinyl chitosan (NSC, a cationic biopolymer derivative of chitosan), poly(acrylamide) and poly(acrylic acid). Acrylamide and acrylic acid are two biocompatible synthetic and anionic monomers. N, N'-methylenebisacrylamide (MBA) and ammonium persulfate (APS) were used as cross-linking agent and initiator respectively. Hydrogels were characterized by Fourier transform spectroscopy (FTIR), X-ray diffraction (XRD) and differential scanning calorimetry (DSC). Hydrogels were synthesized by varying the concentration of monomer, initiator and crosslinking agent. Percentage yield, gel content and gel time were examined, and excellent results were found. This study revealed that the latter, were significantly affected by varying the concentration of monomers, initiator and cross-linking agent. In addition, their hydrogel was thermally stable with a highly porous network and novel rheological characteristics. Theophylline encapsulated in this hydrogel system, which targets the colon to release this active substance, improves respiration. Furthermore, it was observed that the efficacy of encapsulation depended on the composition of the hydrogel. The theophylline release study revealed that the rate of release varied according to the pH and composition of the hydrogel. Maximum release was 24% and 93% in buffer solutions of pH 1.2 and 7.4, respectively. Release kinetics followed an anomalous non-Fickian transport mechanism (good fit to the Ritger-Peppas model) and theophylline maintained its chemical activity after in vitro release. Bashir et al. used N,N'-methylenebisacrylamide as a cross-linking agent, as it is biocompatible with the human body. Formaldehyde, glutaraldehyde and tripolyphosphate are among the cross-linking agents available on the market, but certain limitations are associated with their use, such as their toxicity and the problem of disposing of unreacted toxic materials after hydrogel manufacture [1].

Wang et al (2017) encapsulated the drugs amoxicillin and meloxicam in a chitosan/poly (acrylic acid) cross-linked hydrogel, thanks to which they obtained three pH-sensitive hydrogels designed to control drug release. To improve drug targeting to the physiologically active site, Wang et al. prepared a chitosan derivative called chitosan-g-maleic anhydride (CSMAH) [2]. Ammonium persulfate (APS) was the initiator and CSMAH was the cross-linking agent, by radical polymerization as Bashir et al. (2017) did with N-succinyl chitosan [1-2]. The swelling behavior of these hydrogels and their swelling time showed that hydrogel swelling depends on the extent of crosslinking and the pH of the solution. Release of amoxicillin and meloxicam was enhanced with increasing pH, but hydrogel binding between hydrogel components and between hydrogel and drugs decreased release. Drug release kinetics followed the Korsemeyer - Peppas and Weibull models. These hydrogels appeared to provide an ideal basis for controlled drug delivery systems. Hydrogel swelling and pore size increased as the extent of cross-linking decreased. Release was ensured by a combination of diffusion and relaxation of the hydrogel [2].

Li et al (2020) constructed a physically and chemically cross-linked poly(acrylamide-co-acrylic)/chitosan hydrogel embedded with chitosan-decorated halloysite nanotubes for exceptional mechanical performance. Unfortunately, conventional polymer hydrogel was a mechanically weak class of materials with low extensibility (< 500%), low mechanical strength (< 0.1 MPa) and limited toughness (< 1.0 MJ. m^{-3}) due to the lack of an effective energy dissipation mechanism. To overcome these shortcomings, efforts have been made to design robust mechanical hydrogels such as double-lattice hydrogels, microsphere composite hydrogels, topological hydrogels and ionically cross-linked hydrogels. Among these are nanocomposite hydrogels, composed of organic and inorganic components; they have been widely studied because of the remarkable improvement in mechanical properties derived from the excellent physico-chemical properties and structure of nanomaterials.

In recent periods, various nanomaterials such as silica nanoparticles, magnetite nanoparticles, montmorillonite, graphene oxide, carbon nanotubes and cellulose crystals have been introduced into the hydrogel network to enhance mechanical performance. Halloysite nanotubes (HNT) are a new natural clay, which has been widely used in interesting applications due to its large surface area, good biocompatibility and low cost. All the existing properties of conventional composite materials indicate that HNTs should be a potential candidate for enhancing the mechanical performance of the hydrogel system.

Li et al. in their study, developed a nanocomposite hydrogel composed of a chemically cross-linked network and an ionically cross-linked network with chitosan-decorated halloysite nanotubes as reinforced nanofillers, which possessed high strength, superior toughness and exceptional extensibility at a water content of 80% by weight.

Meanwhile, mechanical performance could be flexibly modulated by adjusting the CS-f-HNT content and soaking time in the $Fe^{3}+$ solution.

What's more, the $Fe^{3}+$-poly(acrylamide-co-acrylic) CS / CS-f-HNTs hydrogel also displayed excellent self-recovery properties under small deformation (200%) or large deformation (1000%) at room temperature. By optimizing the matrix components, the final nanocomposite hydrogel containing 80 wt.% water content exhibited never-before-reported results, including superior tensile strength (3.06 MPa), high extensibility (2015%) and ultra-high toughness (47.6 MJ/m^3). Li et al. obtained the hydrogel by a facile two-step method consisting of in situ free-radical polymerization and an ion quenching strategy. Hyperbranched vinyl group polysiloxane (HSiv) was the crosslinker and APS the initiator. Radical polymerization was carried out at 45°C for 24 hours. The hydrogels prepared were immersed in a 0.3 M Fe^{3+} solution for a period of time at room temperature [3].

Cao et al (2020) synthesized a physically cross-linked double hydrogel (DPC) based on chitosan and poly (acrylic acid), chitosan/poly (acrylamide-co-acrylic acid) and chitosan/poly (acrylonitrile-co-acrylic acid). Firstly, complex polyelectrolyte hydrogels (PECs) were prepared by in situ polymerization of acrylic acid monomers in chitosan solutions. Subsequently, multivalent cations and anions were introduced into PEC hydrogels to form strong electrostatic interactions with polymer chains, in order to obtain DPC hydrogels. Radical polymerization between chitosan and acrylic acid was engineered at 60°C for 24 h. The unique structure (CS : AAc = 1 : 2.5 the optimum ratio between chitosan and acrylic acid) and the strong interaction between the polymer chains enhanced the mechanical properties of the DPC hydrogels. Furthermore, due to the colligative property of ionic compounds, such as CaCl2 to lower the freezing point of the aqueous phase, the DPC hydrogels of Cao et al. could retain their extensibility and conductivity at -20°C and displayed high, linear stretch sensitivity over a wide stress range, making them suitable as antifreeze sensors in sub-zero environments. With environmental impact, health hazards and low cost in mind, antifreeze hydrogels containing inorganic salts have been attracting more attention recently.

Compared with PEC hydrogels, the DPC method endowed hydrogels with a unique internal structure and excellent mechanical properties. Electrostatic interactions distributed throughout the hydrogels could serve as "sacrificial bonds" to dissipate energy. The mechanical properties of DPC hydrogels increased with increasing ionic concentration and valence state of the loading ions. Trivalent cations showed a much more powerful crosslinking capacity than di- and monovalent cations due to their strong affinity for the carboxyl groups of poly (acrylic acid). Double hydrogels physically cross-linked with Ca^{2+} cations demonstrated stable electrical conductivity and stable sensitivity to tensile stress and temperature, which could be used in antifreeze sensors, actuators and wearable devices [4].

Tanveer et al (2021) prepared biodegradable superabsorbent hydrogels (SAH), derived from chitosan and acrylic acid, crosslinked with vinyltrimethoxysilane (VTMS). The VTMS cross-linking agent was used to promote water uptake and retention capacity of the prepared hydrogels. Variable amounts of alumina nanoparticles (Al NPs) were incorporated into the HSAs.

Tanveer et al. characterized the SAHs with FTIR, SEM, antibacterial activity analysis, soil burial degradation analysis and swelling analysis. Results indicated that all hydrogels were biodegradable. Hydrogels containing 0.08 g of alumina nanoparticles (the maximum concentration of Al NPs used in their study) showed the fastest degradation, within 10 days, while SAHs with a lower concentration of Al NPs were completely degraded within 15 days. The swelling rate of HSAs increased as the concentration of Al NPs increased. Knowing that chitosan was used as a water-absorbing agent, and that acrylic acid has the ability to gel and form a hydrogel with superabsorbent properties, as it is a hydrophilic monomer.

Acrylic acid can be polymerized in the presence of light, heat and peroxides. Applications include superabsorbent hydrogels, paints, textiles, drug delivery and cosmetics. Grafting acrylic acid onto natural polymers enhances the hydrogel's biodegradability. Being pH-sensitive and inherently biodegradable, these HSAs have proven to be smart materials that tend to increase soil porosity and provide more pathways for water transport in semi-arid, arid and desert areas. The SAHs developed showed good swelling in both acidic and basic environments due to the presence of acidic (AAc) and basic (CS) groups. The SAHs synthesized by Tanveer et al. showed exceptional antimicrobial properties. Thanks to their eco-benign nature, their use can be extended to other fields, such as biomedicine [5].

Jiang et al (2021) succeeded in preparing a nanocomposite organohydrogel achieving good mechanical properties and high tolerance to hot and cold environments, which remains a recent challenge. In their work, Jiang et al. introduced ethylene glycol (EG) and cellulose (CNF) nanofibrils into chitosan/poly(acrylamide-acrylic acid) dual network hydrogels, to improve their toughness and tolerance to hot and cold environments. EG increased the hydrogel's tolerance to hot and cold environments. However, EG had a negative effect on the hydrogels' mechanical properties. In addition, CNFs significantly improved the strength of chitosan/poly (acrylamide-acrylic acid)/EG organohydrogels. Jiang et al. offer a new route to preparing high-strength, tough organohydrogels with high tolerance to hot and cold environments. Their method appears to be a practical solution for transporting and storing organohydrogels [6].

II.6.3. **Conclusion**

It was noted that acrymide acid always accompanies acrylic acid in chitosan-based composite blends. Despite the use of radical polymerization, incorporating acrylic acid and acrymide acid into the chitosan matrix, the hydrogel remained a highly physical bionanocomposite with mechanical drawbacks.

Methods such as soaking the hydrogel in a mineral solution, or intercalating mineral nanofillers in the polymer melt (one-pot method), provide a kind of antiseptic hydrogel capable of controlled release of antibacterial agents, improved swelling and toughness, and the ability to remain flexible at very low temperatures. The addition of cellulose or halloysite nanofibers, and the use of CS derivatives (pre-treated CS) with their specific cross-linking agent, may become necessary to improve the resistance during storage and transport of hydrogels, defined in the latter case, as a chemical bionanocomposite hydrogel.

References

[1] . S. Bashir, Y.-Y. Teo, S. Ramesh, K. Ramesh. Physico-chemical characterization of pH- sensitive N-Succinyl chitosan-g-poly (acrylamide-co-acrylic acid) hydrogels and in vitro drug release studies. Polymer degradation and Stability, 139 (2017) 38-54.

[2] . Y. Wang, J. Wang, Z. Yuan, H. Han, T. Li, L. Li, X. Guo. Chitosan cross-linked poly(acrylic acid) hydrogels: Drug release control and mechanism. Colloids and Surfaces B: Biointerfaces, 152 (2017) 252-259.

[3] . S.-N. Li, B. Li, Z.-R. Yu, Y. Li, K.-Y. Guo, L.-X. Gong, Y. Feng, D. Jia, Y. Zhou, L.-C. Tang. Constructing dual ionically cross-linked poly(acrylamide-co-acrylic acid)/chitosan hydrogel materials embedded with chitosan decorated halloysite nanotubes for exceptional mechanical performance. Composites Part B 194 (2020) 108 046.

[4] . J. Cao, Y. Wang, C. He, Y. Kang, J. Zhou. Ionically crosslinked chitosan/poly(acrylic acid) hydrogels with high strength, toughness and antifreezing capability. Carbohydrate Polymers 242 (2020) 116 420.

[5] . M. Tanveer, A. Farooq, S. Ata, I. Bibi, M. Sultan, M. Iqbal, S. Jabeen, N. Gull, A. Islam, R.-U. Khan, S.-H. Al Mijalli. Aluminum nanoparticles, chitosan, acrylic acid and vinyltrimethoxysilane based hybrid hydrogel as a remarkable water super-absorbent and antimicrobial activity, Surfaces and Interfaces, 25 (2021) 101 285.

[6] . Z. Jiang, L. Guo, F. Yuan, J. Wang, X. Jiang. Tough chitosan/poly(acrylamide-acrylic acid)/cellulose nanofibrils/ ethylene glycol nanocomposite organohydrogel with tolerance to hot and cold environments, International Journal of biological Macromolecules, 186 (2021) 952-961.

[7] . M. Gandi, H. Zemmouri, M. Amari. Research on bionanocomposites of therapeutic value: Bio and hydro-engineering nano-molecular organic oligo engineering. February 10, 2021, LibroWorld, ISBN-10: 6203313351/ ISBN-13: 9786203313352, 60 p.

Chapter 7: Carbon Dioxide Hazard in Liquid and Semi-Solid Oral Pharmaceutical Forms.

11.7.1. Foreword

It has been discovered that the presence of carbon dioxide in the atmosphere generates aqueous bicarbonate ions by transforming aqueous hydroxyl ions. These ions act as toxins for the human body when introduced with the drug. The best atmospheric parameter to control when manufacturing liquid/semi-solid oral dosage forms, other than temperature and pressure, residual air humidity or air filtration to remove dust, is the carbon dioxide concentration, to ensure the best bioavailability and least toxicity for these prepared dosage forms, in polluted industrial areas.

11.7.2. Bibliographic research

Due to the dissolution of atmospheric carbon dioxide in water, bicarbonate ions are produced in chemical solutions, the latter ions being the conjugate base of aqueous carbon dioxide, a weak acid. Bicarbonate ions are responsible for the alkalinity of water, as aqueous hydroxyl ions are converted to bicarbonate ions by aqueous carbon dioxide, and thus the pH of water rises above 7 [1]. In view of this finding, the presence of atmospheric carbon dioxide must be eliminated in workshops manufacturing liquid/semi-solid oral forms of drugs, as the bicarbonate ions generated by aqueous carbon dioxide have adverse consequences for the infiltration of drugs into the body. The administration of bicarbonate into the extracellular space is associated with a number of potentially serious adverse effects, in particular hypokalemia, and can actually exacerbate intracellular acidosis. Bicarbonate ions (which cannot diffuse through cell membranes) combine extracellularly with H+ ions, producing carbonic acid which dissociates into water and carbon dioxide. The latter easily penetrates cells, where the reverse reaction occurs, generating H+ (and bicarbonate) ions intracellularly. This also generates paradoxical acidosis of the cerebrospinal fluid, and adverse effects on the oxyhaemoglobin dissociation curve (leftward shift of the oxyhaemoglobin dissociation curve, which alters the release of oxygen from haemoglobin to tissues in the event of low cardiac output and low oxygen supply [3]), as well as excessive alkalosis (these are other adverse effects). Concerns have also been expressed about the potential for accelerating ketogenesis (and lactate generation (the latter produces cramps, muscle aches or pains [5])) by increasing pH with bicarbonate [2].

Note: Ketogenesis is a metabolic process essential to life, enabling survival under fasting conditions. In the event of a sugar deficit, this pathway leads to the formation of ketone bodies, which are transported to the brain to provide energy instead of glucose [4].

References

[1] . W. Bleam, 2017. Soil and Environnmental Chemistry (Second Edition). Chapter 6- AcidBase Chemistry. Page 253-331.

[2] . S. Ghosh, A. Collier, 2012. Section 4- Acute metabolic complications. Churchill's Pocketbook of diabetes (Second Edition). Pages 127-164.

[3] . J. M. Schwartz, E. S. Heitmiller, E. A. Hunt, D. H. Shaffner, 2011. Chapter 38- Cardiopulmonary Resuscitation. Smith's Anesthesia for Infants and Childern (Eighth Edition). Pages 1200-1249.

[4] . https://nutrixeal-info.fr ' index ' cetogenese.

[5] . https://www.cairn.info ' revue-staps-2001-1-page-63.

Chapter 8: Synthesis of Bionanocomposites, with Antiseptic Effects on the Skin, in the Absence, of Systematic Obstruction in Empirical Trials.

Introduction Chapter 8

The engineering of new materials with therapeutic applications is a major engineering outcome of biomedicine. For this purpose, nanotechnology has innovated nanomaterials with excellent physicochemical properties, inducing a higher rate of efficacy, and a wider spread over the surface, compared to the volume, of the bulk product. These nanomaterials can be divided into two groups, organic or inorganic, depending on their source of derivation. Take, for example, the metals Ag, Cu, and their metal oxides CuO, $Ag_2 O$.

Recently, the medicinal and industrial importance of nanoparticles has gained more consideration. However, metal NPs can be cytotoxic under human physiological conditions, as well as hazardous to the environment. This problem has been resolved by recent investigations using various methods, such as :

- Encapsulation of metal NPs.
- Incorporation of metal NPs.
- Loading with metal NPs.

To overcome the problem of biocompatibility and biodegradability in hydrogels, composites and films, various synthetic and natural materials play a complementary role. The most widely used natural polymers are polysaccharides such as chitosan, cellulose and alginate, which attract more attention than other polymers for their abundance and benign effects on the human body and the environment. Coupling these polymers with metal NPs or metal oxides can enhance their therapeutic effects. The four stages of dermal wound healing:

- Hemostasis.
- Inflammation.
- Proliferation.
- Remodeling.

It should be emphasized that the bottle containing the bulk product plays an important role in the success of each stage of wound healing. In addition, the anti-bacterial capacity of metal nanoparticles as antibacterial agents can be modified by changing the size and morphology of the nanoparticles. The smaller the size of metal nanoparticles, the better they are at getting rid of bacteria, while diversifying the morphology of metal nanoparticles, e.g. spherical or tubular, improves their anti-bacterial activity compared with a uniform shape (Alavi et al., 2020). Among the modern dressings produced in recent years, films, foams, hydrocolloids, sponges and hydrogels are the most popular. But, hydrogels, are the preferred ones, thanks to their moist nature, which hydrates, the wound bed, and their gain capabilities in the quantity of the final product, following their swelling affinities, 10 times more, than the initial quantity, with distilled water alone (Joorabloo et al., 2018).

References

Alavi, M.; Nokhodchi, A., An overview on antimicrobial and wound healing properties of ZnO nanobiofilms, hydrogels, and bionanocomposites based on cellulose, chitosan, and alginate polymers. Carbohydrate Polymers 227 (2020) 115349.

Joorabloo, A.; Khorasani, M.T.; Adeli, H.; Mansoori-Moghadam, Z.; Moghaddam, A., Fabrication of Heparinized Nano ZnO/ Poly(vinylalcohol)/ Carboxymethyl Cellulose Bionanocomposite Hydrogels using Artificial Neural Network for Wound Dressing Application. JOURNAL OF INDUSTRIAL AND ENGINEERING CHEMISTRY. 2018.

II.8.1. **Zinc oxide**

The controlled release of Zn 2+ ions from zinc oxide particles (ZnO NPs), coupled with natural polymers such as cellulose, chitosan and alginate, in the form of nanocomposites, should be an indispensable parameter for obtaining suitable industrial formulations for modern, healthy and cost-effective scaffolds used for wound healing. The side effects of ZnO/chitosan, ZnO/cellulose and ZnO/alginate systems are quite tolerable, so these systems have gained more attention in physiological applications.

The functional groups, hydroxyls and amines of cellulose and chitosan, accessible to interact, are responsible for their negligible cytotoxicities. In addition to this mechanism, ZnO NPs can form reactive oxygen species under certain wavelengths of light (ultraviolet and visible light). This last mechanism provides porous hydration, which increases the suitability, biocompatibility and biodegradability of these ZnO NPs, compared with other metal NPs, in the therapeutic and cosmetic fields, towards humans, not forgetting their ecosystem. Let's not forget that zinc oxide nanoparticles are trace elements that act against physiological bacterial microorganisms, especially eukaryotic and prokaryotic microorganisms.

With regard to their antimicrobial, anticancer, antidiabetic and wound-healing properties, the oligodynamic activities of ZnO NPs have been widely reported. In fact, ZnO NPs damage nucleic acid and bacterial expression genes, thanks to the presence of reactive oxygen species. This phenomenon can be observed at the biomacromolecular level (Alavi et al. 2020). Zinc oxide nanoparticles can be synthesized in a number of ways, including precipitation, soaking, sol-gel transition (reversible transformation from liquid suspension to gel by temperature reduction or pH increase), solid-state pyrolysis (thermal melting), and green chemistry (no toxic products for humans or the environment). Molecularly modified ZnO NPs, produced in gel form with (3 glycidyloxypropyl) trimethoxysilane, showed increased anti-bacterial activity against E. coli, despite the rise in temperature, for quite some time (600°C, 24 h).

High-energy ball milling is a large-scale, physical milling process that produces chips (fragments) of solid ZnO nanoparticles. The high-energy ball milling method offers advantages such as simplicity, reproducibility and well-controlled size and shape. The longer the milling time, the more the ZnO NPs shrink, guaranteeing better bactericidal activity. Molecular docking (molecular anchoring), a computational molecular tool, has been of great help to scientists in this context. ZnO NPs are known to target the outer membrane of bacteria such as E. Coli (Alavi et al., 2020). The latter, phenomenon is monitored , in the presence of an NMR spectrometer: solid-state nuclear magnetic resonance, which provides a spectroscopic tool for deducing structure and biodynamicity across the lipid bilayer, at the level of proteins constituting bacterial membranes, and more recently, in the environment surrounding the bacteria (Pinto et al., 2018), thanks to the formation of H-bridges between ZnO NPs and residues of the amino acid asparagine, a compound of the protein barrier in the bacterial outer membrane. The dipping method is a chemical approach to the manufacture of metal NPs, which depends on the type of metal salt and other precursors, as well as on the concentration of each reagent and the temperature. These factors directly influence the size and morphology of metal nanoparticles, i.e. their physicochemical properties (Alavi et al., 2020). Zinc oxide nanoparticles are non-toxic, distribute evenly in the polymer matrix, spread easily on the skin, as well as possessing long-term stability, degrading with difficulty in moist environments. This makes ZnO NPs a promising anti-bacterial component in localized skin dressing materials (Masud et al., 2020).

References

Alavi, M.; Nokhodchi, A., An overview on antimicrobial and wound healing properties of ZnO nanobiofilms, hydrogels, and bionanocomposites based on cellulose, chitosan, and alginate polymers. Carbohydrate Polymers 227 (2020) 115349.

Pinto, C.; Mance, D; Sinnige, T.; Daniels, M.; Weingarth, M.; & Baldus, M., Formation of the β-barrel assembly machinery complex in lipid bilayers as seen by solid-state NMR. Nature Communications volume 9, Article number: 4135 (2018).

Masud, R.A. ; Islam, Md. S.; Haque, P.; I Khan, M.N.; Shahruzzaman, Md.; Khan, M.; Takafuji, M.; Rahman, Md.M., Preparation of novel chitosan/poly (ethylene glycol)/ZnO bionanocomposite for wound healing application: Effect of gentamicin loading. Materialia 000 (2020) 100785.

II.8.2. **Cellulose**

Cellulose is a natural, renewable biodegradable polymer. It is widely distributed in plant cells and certain aquatic organisms, and is even generated by microbial biosynthesis (bacteria, algae, fungi) (Vijayakumar et al., 2021). This macromolecule has three hydroxyl groups in each monomer, which are accessible for interaction with chemical substrates, making it easy to modify. This molecular modification approach aims to improve the wound dressing materials produced, whether as a local medicine (bionanocomposite hydrogel), or a medical device (a block bionanocomposite = structural bionanocomposite, or solid scaffold bionanocomposite), in biomedical applications for the cure of wounds (Alavi et al., 2020).

To obtain appropriate physicochemical properties, the nanotechnological facet of this polysaccharide must be taken into consideration. The nanoforms of cellulose are :

- Cellulose nanofibrils (NFC).
- Nanocrystalline cellulose (NCC) (Alavi et al., 2020).

As these cellulose nanoforms alone are not sufficient for better healing, biochemical modifications are currently required, such as the incorporation of cellulose/keratin nanofibrils into a natural tragacanth hydrogel, which has been shown to be more effective at healing (Alavi et al., 2020). The cellulose- NPs Ag system has shrunk the size of the noble metal nanoparticles obtained, rounding them down to between 50 and 100 nm, thus ensuring uniform distribution and optimum consistency in pharmaceutical forms for topical applications. Functionalized nano-crystallites are the only raw material suitable for use in bionanocomposite hydrogels, which is also a powerful bactericidal agent against infected skin cells, whether ordinary or cancerous (proven on breast cancer in vitro), according to a recent study. The green synthesis of cellulose nanocrystallites-NPs Ag-is a vital method for creating an environment in which humans can live in a healthy, unpolluted environment (Vijayakumar et al., 2021).

References

Vijayakumar, S.; Chen, J.; Amarnath, M.; Tungare, K.; Bhori, M.; Divya,M.; Gonzalez- Shanchez, Z.I.; Duran-Lara, E.F.; Vaseeharan, B., Cytotoxicity, phytotoxicity, and photocatalytic assessment of biopolymer cellulose-mediated silver nanoparticles. Colloids and Surfaces A: Physicochemical and Engineering Aspects, 628 (2021) 127170.

Alavi, M.; Nokhodchi, A., An overview on antimicrobial and wound healing properties of ZnO nanobiofilms, hydrogels, and bionanocomposites based on cellulose, chitosan, and alginate polymers. Carbohydrate Polymers 227 (2020) 115349

II.8.3. **Chitosan**

Chitosan, the deacetylated product of chitin, is a cationic biopolymer, which has been used as a matrix for bio-nanocomposites with a range of nano-reinforcements such as clays, chitin and cellulose nanofibrils.

In recent times, there has been immense interest in producing organic-inorganic nanocomposite hydrogels because of their biomedical significance: various nanocomposite hydrogels are considered suitable drug carriers, since they often exhibit extremely better properties than pure polymer hydrogels. The addition of nanoparticles, whether organic or inorganic, to polymeric matrices can reduce the bursting effect of drug release, improve stability and offer slower or more constant release of bionanocomposite drugs.

According to the literature, inorganic NPs added to chitosan nanocomposites are montmorillonite NPs, attapulgite NPs, hydroxyapatite NPs, palygorskite NPs, vermiculite NPs, etc. (Zafar at al., 2016). Silver nanoparticles, Ag NPs, are less preferred, compared to zinc oxide NPs, in antimicrobial products, due to their mild toxicities, despite their higher antibacterial activities (Zafar at al. 2016; Gandi at al., 2022). However, silver nanoparticles are still used in clothing, medical devices, cosmetics and pharmaceuticals. This is due to their distinctive physico-chemical and anti-bacterial properties. They guarantee a higher swelling capacity in chitosan hydrogels than in pure chitosan hydrogels (Zafar et al., 2016).

References

Zafar, R.; Zia, K.M.; Tabasum, S.; Jabeen, F.; Noreen, A.; Zuber, M., Polysaccharide based bionanocomposites, properties and applications: A review. International Journal of Biological Macromolecules, 92 (2016) 1-13.

Gandi, M.; Benabdelghani, Z.; Amari, M., paperback: bionanocomposites in the biomedical industry (2nd edition), Decitre, Éditions Universitaires Européennes, ISBN: 978-613-846469-3. 80 pgs. 2022.

II.8.4. Collagen

Biopolymer nanocomposites can be used in dentistry, biomedical tissue engineering, and human bone repair or replacement. The main use for bionanocomposites, however, is in local dressings, with a well-studied delivery system and anti-microbial properties that are non-toxic, non-corrosive and free of recorded side effects, not to mention their ability to maintain a moist, healthy bed on infected skin beds, leaving no post-treatment eschar. Zinc oxide particles require fewer quantities and doses to be introduced into a biomedical product formula in the form of dressings (with all its phases of final constituent material), compared with the dose of other metals that would be chosen to incorporate alone into a formula, as antibacterial agents that bring about ideal, much-sought-after healing.

Collagen, as the most abundant, biocompatible protein and a biodegradable material, is extracted from various animal tissues and could be used in a wide range of biomedical applications. Among collagen's applications are its bionanocomposite films, functionalized with ZnO NPs, which act as a high-performance protective barrier on the skin against UV rays, preventing corrosivity and enhancing hydration. That said, ZnO NPs are the components that improve these parameters compared with ZnO NP-free films. These films are competitive products for wound-healing and biosensing systems (Mallakpour et al., 2021).

References

Mallakpour, S.; Sirous, F.; Hussain, C.M., A journey to the world of fascinating ZnO nanocomposites made of chitosan, starch, cellulose, and other biopolymers: Progress in recent achievements in eco-friendly food packaging, biomedical, and water remediation technologies. International Journal Of Biomacromolecules, 170 (2021) 701-716.

Gentamicin, a natural aminoglycoside, is an antibiotic whose therapeutic effects, in topical galenic forms, is the treatment of minor skin infections ([*]). In a recent study (2020), the antibacterial bionanocomposite system consisted of a mixture of zinc oxide nanoparticles (ZnO NPs) and two polymers, one natural, chitosan (CS), and the other synthetic, poly(ethylene glycol) (PEG), all cross-linked by sodium tripolyphosphate (STPP), with Gentamicin stored in the matrix. The bionanocomposite obtained by the mixing and shaping processes exhibited a controlled and prolonged delivery of bioactive substances, with a mutual and enhanced bactericidal effect, as a result of the compensation, at wound-healing level, between the antibacterial agents, i.e. ZnO NPs, and Gentamicin. This CS/ PEG/ ZnO NPs system, cross-linked by STPP and purified by NaOH, is a potential basic candidate as a topical cargo system for anti-bacterial active substances (Masud et al., 2020).

The bionanocomposite in the form of hemostatic gauze, defined as a sticky dressing soaked with a compound that stops bleeding, in the study described above, consisting of CS/PEG/NPs ZnO/STPP loaded with Gentamicin, gave better wound-healing results in vivo than hemostatic gauze without Gentamicin, which in turn was better than conventional medical gauze, defined therapeutically as dry bandage gauze (Masud et al. 2020).

In their study, Masud et al. mixed solutions of chitosan dissolved in acetic acid using a magnetic stirrer, incorporating prefabricated nanoparticles of PEG and then ZnO, while sodium tripolyphosphate was added last. A white precipitate of the composite mixture was observed when the solution was neutralized with 1 M sodium hydroxide.

The precipitate was separated by centrifugation at 5000 rpm for 10 min and washed with distilled water until the pH reached 7 (Masud et al. 2020). Centrifugation is a process for separating the constituents of a mixture on the basis of density difference. Colloidal particles settle out, leaving the less dense particles to float on top ([**]).

The best mechanical properties of the bionanocomposite (better stability, flexibility and high porosity) were obtained with a STPP:CS mass ratio of 0.3:1. For other, lower or higher STPP:CS ratios, the wet bionanocomposite sheets were too hard and brittle.

On the other hand, the drug solution, based on Gentamicin sulfate, at very low concentrations, in contact with the bionanocomposite foils, CS/PEG/NPs ZnO/STPP, was shaken in an orbital shaker (Masud et al. 2020), also known as an orbital mixer or shaker or laboratory reciprocator, a device used for extraction processes ([***]), at 110 rpm for 24 h at room temperature, to facilitate gentamicin uptake (and in our opinion probably homogeneously). The percentage loading efficiency of the active substance was calculated. Loading efficiency is defined as the ratio between the initial drug concentration in the initial soaking liquid and the concentration of unreacted drug remaining in the supernatant liquid after soaking the sample at the initial drug concentration, as follows (Masud et al. 2020):

Loading efficiency

$$= \frac{\text{concentration initiale}_{\text{médicament}} - \text{concentration dans le surnageant}_{\text{médicament}}}{\text{concentration initiale}_{\text{médicament}}} \times 100$$

References

Masud, R.A.; Islam, Md.S.; Haque, P.; I Khan, M.N.; Shahruzzaman, Md.; Khan, M.; Takafuji, M.; Rahman, Md.M., Preparation of novel chitosan/poly (ethylene glycol)/ZnO bionanocomposite for wound healing application: Effect of gentamicin loading. Materialia 000 (2020) 100785.

[*]. https://www.advacarepharma.com/fr/medicaments/pommade-de-gentamicine.

[**]. https://fr.wikipedia.org/wiki/Centrifugation.

[***]. https://fr.vwr.com/store/product/596014/melangeur-secoueur-orbital-ou-va-et vient-de- laboratoire-ssl2.

II.8.6. **Heparin**

Heparin is a natural macromolecule produced by human immune cells, making up 30% of human body tissue. This active ingredient, treats thrombosis, blood clotting, in the form of clots (Colllot, 2015). Forms of thrombosis include: cutaneous arteriolar thrombosis (Figure 17), also known as superficial venous thrombosis, or superficial thrombophlebitis (Jeanneret-Gris et al., 2006), and stasis dermatitis (Figure 18), also known as stasis dermatitis, or venous stasis, which can be considered one of the types of superficial venous thrombosis, among others ([*1]; Carsuzaa et al., 2002). Both diseases are caused by blood clotting and water retention (Jeanneret-Gris et al., 2006, Ruenger, 2023, [*2]). However, its production on an industrial scale is derived from animal cells, and this is what led to fatal deaths by intravenous injection and hundreds of allergic reactions to local forms in 2002, from production in China to Germany and the USA, and it was under these circumstances that scientists began to produce biosynthesized heparin enzymatically ([*3]). Enzymes are produced by fermenting living microorganisms in a fermenter, and this is the method for their large-scale synthesis, as opposed to extraction from plant or animal cells ([*4]).

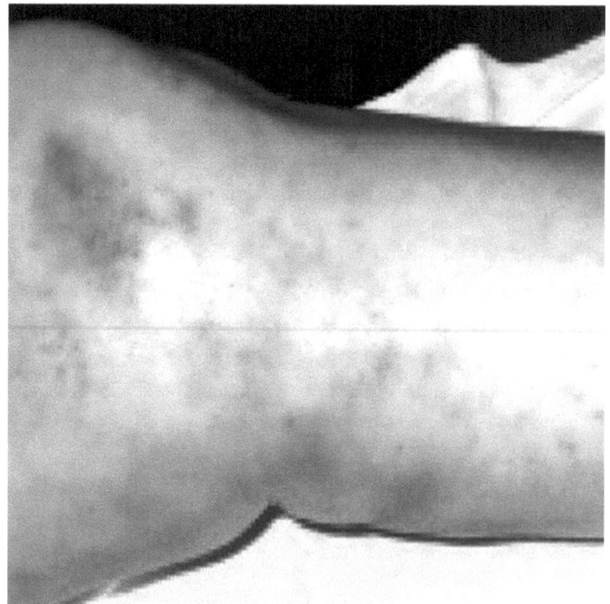

Figure 17. Superficial cutaneous thrombosis (Jeanneret-Gris et al., 2006).

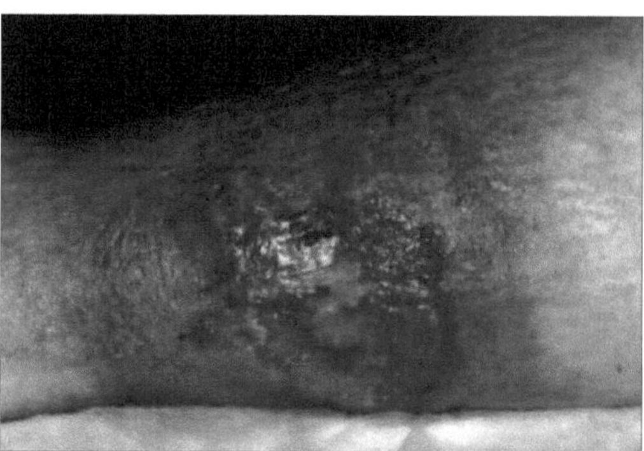

Figure 18. Stasis dermatitis (Ruenger, 2023).

Heparin, with an absorption peak at 556 nm in the UV-visible, in a buffer solution, of methylene blue, improved the anti-bacterial bioactivity of an antibacterial bionanocomposite hydrogel, compared with the hydrogel without heparin, based on ZnO NPs, and two synthetic polymers CMC (carboxymethylcellulose) and PVA (polyvinyl acetate).

The components of the composite mixture were mixed for 1 h, first in a homogenizer, then for a further 8 h, on a magnetic mixer. Joorabloo et al. (2018), subjected, the hydrogels, to 3 freeze-thaw cycles, placing them at -20°C, or room temperature, and vice versa. At the end, the hydrogel was freeze-dried, for 24 h, for better porosity. According to the data in this study, the hydrogel dressings showed a better state of equilibrium in terms of the degree of swelling after drying, and in terms of the rate of hydration of the infection bed in the skin (WVTR: water vapor transmission rate), this equilibrium having reached the end point with mass percentages of 64.672 $(W_0)\%$, 34.492 $(W_0)\%$ and 0.836 $(W_T)\%$ for PVA, CMC and ZnO NPs.

Heparin was added to the aqueous solution of ZnO NPs according to a specific procedure, before being mixed with the polymer solutions. Infrared analysis showed that the bridges between the heparin molecules and the ZnO NPs were purely physical, but the functionalized polymer matrices appeared to have good mechanical properties, as cited in this manuscript, protecting the hydrogel product from attack by environmental factors around the treated wound.

The higher the dose of ZnO NPs or CMC, the more brittle the hydrogel became. On the other hand, increasing the dose of PVA fortified the hydrogel's mechanical properties, while making it more flexible, due to the smaller size of the PVA crystallites, which had been hybridizing since delivery from the supplier (Joorabloo et al., 2018).

In the interesting study, by Joorabloo et al. (2018), all the extensibilities (elongations at breaking points) obtained from the hydrogels, were low ("500%), and not modernized (like those of the weak, banal mechanical properties of conventional hydrogels, of the past), however, the ultimate tensile strengths, also called, tenacities, were optimized to the minimum acceptable (they were equal to 1 MPa, or higher and close to 1 MPa).

The hydrogel's extensibility and tenacity values, according to our synthetic spirit, in this study, have two obvious meanings: advantageous and disadvantageous, respectively. There is likely to be some deficiency in the therapeutic effect of topical hydrogels, as a result of impeded spreading and penetration on and into the infected skin bed, according to modern extensibility standards. Storing the product in its resting state in the packaging tube (usually made of aluminum), and extracting the desired quantity when used by the patient, will however be easy (Joorabloo et al., 2018; Gandi et al., 2022).

References

Collot, F.; Le guide des médicaments, in Notre temps magazine: Heparin, a molecule against thrombosis. 2015.

Jeanneret-Gris, C.; Baldi, T.; Jenelten, R., Superficial thrombophlebitis: an overview. Swiss Medical Forum, ReaserchGate. 2006.

https://www.veterans.gc.ca/fra/health-support/physical-health-and-wellness/compensation-illness-injury/disability-benefits/benefits-determined/entitlement-eligibility guidelines/varicose#condition2: [*1].

Carouzaa, F. ; Boyo, T., ; Fournier, B. ; Guennoc, G., Thrombose cutanée artériolaire à type de dermite purpuriqueet pigmentaire révélant la mutation G/A 20210 du gène de la prothrombine, LA REVUE DE MEDECINE INTERNE, Elsevier Masson SAS. 2002.

Ruenger, T.M., Stasis dermatitis. THE MERCK MANUAL: Version for health professionals. 2023.

[*2]. https://www.larousse.fr/encyclopedie/medical/ edema/14886.

[*3]. https://www.sciencesetavenir.fr/sante/vers-une-heparine-sans-risques_23796.

https://www.uvt.rnu.tn/resources-uvt/cours/genie_biocatalyse/module1/co/Contenu_07.html: [*4].

Joorabloo, A.; Khorasani, M.T.; Adeli, H.; Mansoori-Moghadam, Z.; Moghaddam, A., Fabrication of Heparinized Nano ZnO/Poly(vinylalcohol)/Carboxymethyl Cellulose Bionanocomposite Hydrogels using Artificial Neural Network for Wound Dressing Application. JOURNAL OF INDUSTRIAL AND ENGINEERING CHEMISTRY. 2018.

Gandi, M.; Benabdelghani, Z.; Amari, M., paperback: bionanocomposites in the biomedical industry (2nd edition), Decitre, Éditions Universitaires Européennes, ISBN: 978-613-846469-3. 80 pgs. 2022.

Nowadays, dressings must enhance the healing process by interacting with the wound, releasing bioactive molecules while preserving the favorable conditions necessary for the restoration of skin integrity and homeostasis. Along with other desired biological properties, polymeric scaffolds need to exhibit improved mechanical strength, stability, skin pore penetration and a well-interconnected intrinsic pore structure. To achieve these critical parameters, the disadvantages associated with synthetic versus natural polymers can be overcome by creating hybrid composite scaffolds based on synthetic polymers with organic/inorganic reinforcements. Natural polymers such as collagen, gelatin, silk fibroin, chitosan, alginate, cellulose and so on are biocompatible and facilitate better interaction with the cells, alive, where the polymerized system is deposited, leading to increased cell proliferation (Masud et al., 2020).

However, biopolymer-only structural composites used to heal infected wounds are impractical, due to their poor mechanical properties and the limited solubility of the compacted biopolymer. This inevitably leads to the addition of inorganic NPs to polymer matrices, so that they play an anti-bacterial role, maintaining the product's biocompatibility and facilitating the dissolution of the wound-healing substance. In order to enhance the antibacterial activities of ZnO NPs, and for the production of suitable nanocomposites, improving electron hopping through the outer layer of these NPs, by adding other metals, is a matter to be taken seriously. Despite the rapid release of antibacterial agents, taking ZnO NPs as an example, the addition of these metal NPs improves the mechanical properties of nanocomposite biopolymers.

There are two problems with galenic formulations where bionanocomposites are loaded with metal NPs: the uncontrollable release of anti-bacterial ions, while a high dose of metal NPs has to be introduced into the formula to avoid side effects, i.e. neutralization of therapeutic effects, but, on the other hand, there is the financial management involved in purchasing a large quantity of raw material at the lowest price. In hydrogels, the release of antibacterial metal ions must be moderate and prolonged. For resolution, the choice of precursor (polymerization initiator) and binding agent is a specific choice, depending on the optimum pH of the formula, the physiological environment concerned, and the ambient temperature of the pharmaceutical product. There are 4 types of hydrogel response, depending on the pH category, to be chosen, for successful healing, to the targeted physiological medium, as follows:

- Polymers with basic physiological response pH.
- Polymers with an acidic physiological pH response.
- Polymers with neutral physiological pH response.
- Polymers with multiple physiological response pH.

The addition of multiple-response synthetic polymers, as a complementary material to the bionanocomposite hydrogel, is now a necessity for a better therapeutic effect. In this context, the bionanocomposite hydrogels NPs ZnO/chitosan, NPs ZnO/cellulose, NPs ZnO/alginate, are complemented by poly[(2-N-morpholino) ethyl methacrylate] (PMEA), and poly-[(2-dimethylaminoethyl) methacrylate] (PDMA) (Alavi et al., 2020). Some researchers have already reported the use of biomedically relevant biopolymers such as chitosan, chitin isolated from Periplaneta americana (American cockroach) wing extract, gelatin, starch, and microcrystalline cellulose, as uniformity dispensers, and as size shrinkers, in the green synthesis, of silver nanoparticles. The green chemistry of silver nanocrystallite production is vital, and eliminates their cytotoxicities, while enhancing their bio-activities, compared to their synthetic manufacture (Vijayakumar et al., 2021). ZnO NPs with their fascinating characteristics could be used to reinforce biopolymer matrices. Globally, they are used for environmentally-friendly food packaging, or as photocatalysts in water purification, not forgetting that they are among the most effective materials in biomedical science (Mallakpour et al., 2021). In conclusion, remember that natural sources of polymers are creating worldwide controversy, despite their biocompatible and non-toxic properties for the human body, as well as their ecological properties towards the environment: polymers obtained directly from nature are more economically valuable on the market (Vijayakumar et al., 2021).

References

Masud, R. A.; Islam, Md. S.; Haque, P.; I Khan, M. N.; Shahruzzaman, Md.; Khan, M.; Takafuji, M.; Rahman, Md. M., Preparation of novel chitosan/poly (ethylene glycol)/ZnO bionanocomposite for wound healing application: Effect of gentamicin loading. Materialia 000 (2020) 100785.

Alavi, M.; Nokhodchi, A., An overview on antimicrobial and wound healing properties of ZnO nanobiofilms, hydrogels, and bionanocomposites based on cellulose, chitosan, and alginate polymers. Carbohydrate Polymers 227 (2020) 115349.

Vijayakumar, S.; Chen, J.; Amarnath, M.; Tungare, K.; Bhori, M.; Divya,M.; Gonzalez- Shanchez, Z.I.; Duran-Lara, E.F.; Vaseeharan, B., Cytotoxicity, phytotoxicity, and photocatalytic assessment of biopolymer cellulose-mediated silver nanoparticles. Colloids and Surfaces A: Physicochemical and Engineering Aspects, 628 (2021) 127170.

Mallakpour, S.; Sirous, F.; Hussain, C.M., A journey to the world of fascinating ZnO nanocomposites made of chitosan, starch, cellulose, and other biopolymers: Progress in recent achievements in eco-friendly food packaging, biomedical, and water remediation technologies. International Journal Of Biomacromolecules, 170 (2021) 701-716.

alginate: salt of alginic acid, an essential constituent of algin, a colorless thickening substance that is difficult to dissolve in water, extracted from certain algae by alkaline treatment.

aminoglycoside: natural plant substance composed of a sugar-based part, in the form of glucosyl groups (these are branches in the form of alkyl units of glucoses (glucose that has lost a hydrogen, to branch with a carbon of a carbon chain)), and also composed of amine functional groups. The main routes of administration for aminoglycosides are intravenous, intramuscular, or topical (external) for the treatment of skin wounds or eye infections, in the form of eye drops.

attapulgite: alumino-magnesian clay with a fibrous morphology, an active anti-inflammatory substance in the form of an oral dressing for the gastrointestinal tract.

loading with metal NPs: re-enforcement of polymer matrix functionalization, by soaking in a saline solution, or by ionotropic dosing.

encapsulation: coating of metal NPs, designed to protect them from external influences, by improving their surface properties, in the materials containing them.

gum tragacanth: synonymous with tracaganth, or dragon's gum, a gummy substance obtained from a variety of small, thorny Asian shrubs of the legume family.

hemostasis: stopping the flow of blood, also known as blood coagulation.

hydroapatite: a mineral compound naturally present in bones and teeth. This bioactive molecule is the main source of calcium and phosphorus in their constitution. Hydroapatite is used in biomedicine for bone and tooth regeneration.

incorporation of metal NPs: condensate homogenization mixing system, in suspension.

inflammation: a set of physiological defense phenomena against an infected aggression, accompanied by pain, redness and swelling.

keratin: this is a group of sulfur-rich proteins, the main constituent of all skin production, from the epidermis in areas of redness, to thin flakes of skin that peel off. Disruption of keratin overproduction in the epidermis is one of the causes of sub-horned pustular dermatosis, a rare skin disease whose symptoms are purulent red or yellow sub-horned pustules and follicular keratoses (rounded, pigmented warts). Other causes of the disease are unknown.

The following figures show the symptoms of subhorn pustular dermatosis.

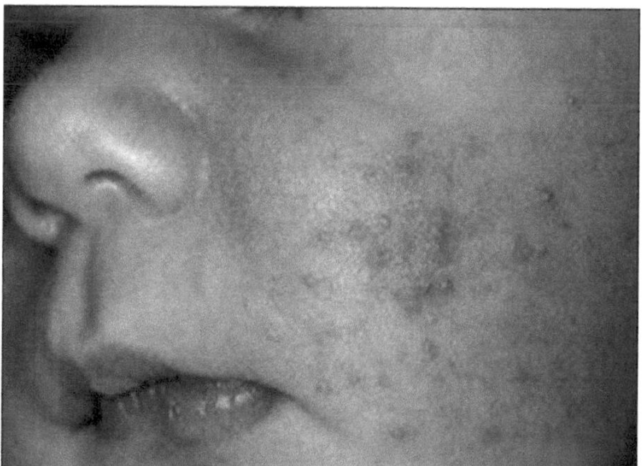

Figure 19. Subcorneal pustules.

Pustules under the horny layer of the skin are called dermatosis pilaris, an overproduction of keratin under the skin, in the pores of the hair growth. The stratum corneum, produced by the epidermis, is an effective, protective, semi-permeable barrier that enables us to survive in the terrestrial environment. It protects against leakage of body fluids, prevents pathogenic compounds from entering the body, and provides a protective barrier against the sun's UV rays. They are initially treated with emollients and moisturizers. This is followed by biotreatment with an oat-based bath. The image of follicular keratosis (horny skin, clogged hair pores) is at bottom right.

Follicular keratoses are a symptom that appears from the age of 50 onwards. Although benign, the disease becomes chronic and intractable. The figure below shows follicular keratosis (horny skin, clogged hair pores).

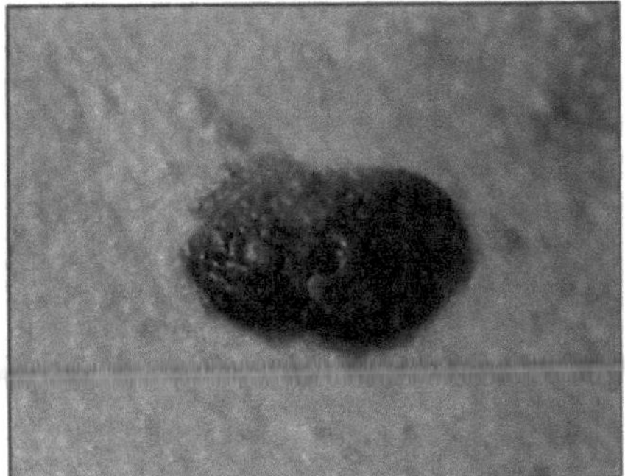
Figure 20. Cutaneous horns.

montmorillonite: n.e., swelling clay mineral, naturally abundant in soils of warm climates, which improves the dry stability of a clay-based paste; it is a plasticizer (degreasing agent).

obstruction: blocking obstacle.

palygorskite: a form of amphibole clay (a mineral based on calcium, magnesium and iron silicates), with a heterogeneous composition, found in eruptive rocks and essentially clayey rocks, the latter known as crystalline schists. The substance is an orally-administered gastrointestinal antibiotic and antidiarrheal.

proliferation: regenerated cells are of incomplete growth.

remodeling: disappearance of infection symptoms and absolute reconstitution of damaged cells.

biosensor system: in biomedicine, this is a medical, analytical, automatic device containing a natural compound, which interacts electro-dynamically with the target physiological substrates, translating the biochemical response by transduction from the sensor, in the form of an electrical signal appearing on its display.

vermiculite: clay mineral, common in tropical zones. Industrially, vermiculite is a thermal insulator in formulas with a high capacity for thickening and texture, swelling under the effect of heat. Vermiculite is used in joint and muscle pain patches to increase their long-lasting effectiveness, and protect them against degradation and damage under the effect of body heat.

Vermiculite is a raw material that can be introduced into the composition of packaging products and hazardous chemical substances, thanks to its anti-corrosive nature; there are other applications for its use, such as: non-degradable anti-corrosion paper, dehydrating bags for cooking, baking, glass-hermetic containers (0 heat transfer), moisture-indicating bags for herbal tea powders.

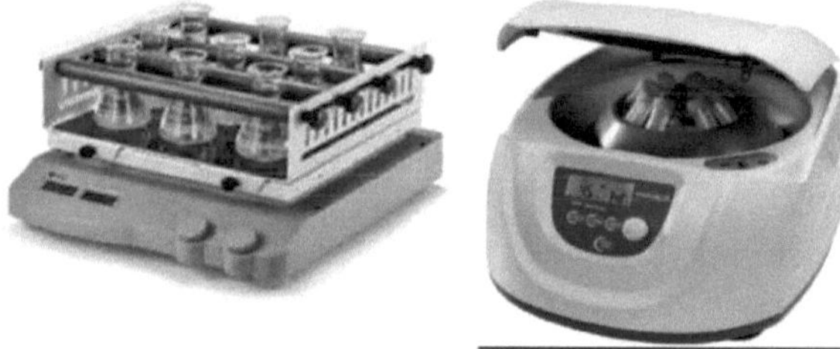

Figure 21. Centrifuge (for solute separation) and orbital homogenizer (for solute extraction), laboratories, from right to left, respectively.

Chapter 9: A Cultivating Passage on Tertiary Bionanocomposite Systems Impregnating Chitosan-Zinc Oxide Nanoparticles-and Other Synthetic or Natural Polymer, in the Decade Prior to 2023.

Introduction Chapter 9

Composite hydrogels as wound dressings offer healing properties in wound treatment. Hydrogel dressings, made from hydrophilic polymers, are used in tissue engineering (functionalization of film dressings), as drug delivery vehicles, or as dressings in their basic states.

Just like film dressings, the water vapor transmission rate (WVTR) is a critical parameter, which concerns lesion hydration. The optimal WVTR in dressing materials is between 2.0-2.5 Kg/m^2/Day. While a high WVTR causes skin dryness and scar formation, a low WVTR leads to the accumulation of exudates in the wound bed and an increase in bacterial growth.

Chitosan (CS) has properties such as high hydrophilicity, biocompatibility, antibacterial activity, gas permeability, moist environment and superior cell adhesion that lead to improved wound healing. The use of zinc oxide (nZnO) nanoparticles in the structure of dressings leads to rapid healing of acute and chronic wounds due to its chemical stability, antibacterial and anti-inflammatory properties, and the release of Zn ions^{2+} next to the wound which leads to increased keratinocyte migration. ZnO nanoparticles have excellent antibacterial biocidal activity, thanks to their large specific surface area. What's more, the US Food and Drug Administration considers ZnO nanoparticles to be safe when exposed to the human body. The cytotoxicity of ZnO nanoparticles is linked to their size and shape. As the size and, logically, the roughness of ZnO nanoparticles decrease, antibacterial and biological activities increase. The concentration below 40 µg/ml is considered non-toxic upon human exposure, for zinc oxide. These bionanocomposite films, especially those with a CS-NPs ZnO mass content ≤ 5.0 wt%, exhibited optimal antibacterial activity, as they were more biocompatible and biodegradable, despite the increase in activity at higher content. Furthermore, the cytotoxicity of ZnO NPs results from the formation of free radicals, also known as reactive oxygen species, on contact with the bacterial cell membrane. This free radical cytotoxicity is the result of a composite mixture, where ZnO molecules are in excess of their maximum solubility, have unpaired electrons, and are hyperactive and very aggressive on physiological tissues. Free radicals can extract electrons from other compounds to achieve stability. In this way, the molecule under attack loses its electron and itself becomes a free radical, triggering a cascade of chain reactions that ultimately damage the living cell. It's up to us, of course, to deduce the development of a superficial tearing of the damaged skin, i.e. skin erosion, the beginning of an ulcer, once developed.

This chapter of the thesis, is a brief, and cultivating, research on bionanocomposite systems, polymerizing zinc oxide chitosan-nanocharges binary systems, by a synthetic or biochemical polymer, respectively, polyvinyl (alcohol), and castor oil, in our choice of wound healing, antibacterial dressings. You'll find two types of dressing in this chapter: hydrogels and films.

References

- Khorasani, M.T.; Joorabloo, A.; Adelib, H.; Mansoori-Moghadam, Z.; Moghaddam, A.. Design and optimization of process parameters of polyvinyl (alcohol)/ chitosan/nano zinc oxide hydrogels as wound healing materials. Carbohydrate Polymers 207 (2019) 542-554.
- Díez-Pascual, A.M.; Díez-Vicente, A.L.. Wound Healing Bionanocomposites Based on Castor Oil Polymeric Films Reinforced with Chitosan-Modified ZnO Nanoparticles. Biomacromolecules 2015, 16, 2631-2644.
- https://www.lanutrition.fr/forme/vieillissement/la-famille-des-radicaux-libres.

Castor oil, also known as castor oil [1], is readily available in nature [2], extracted from castor plant seeds [1], or more rarely from the genital and pre-anal parts of the beaver rodent [3].

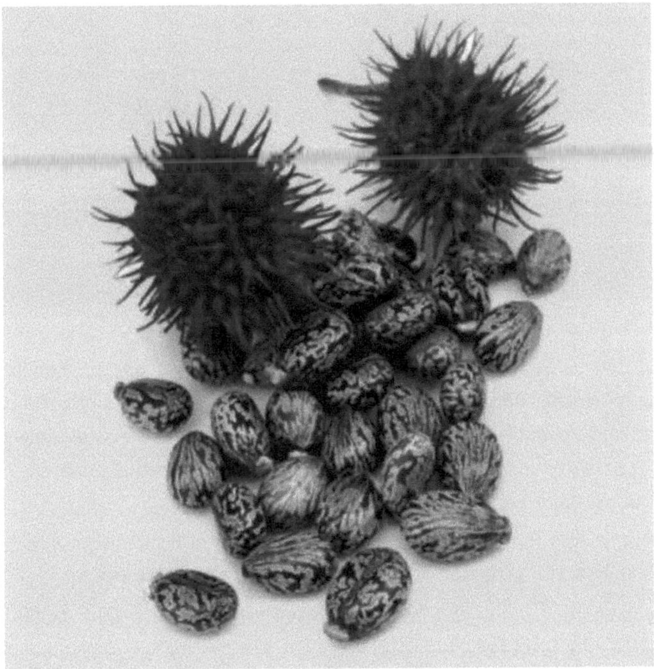
Figure 22. Castor beans [4].

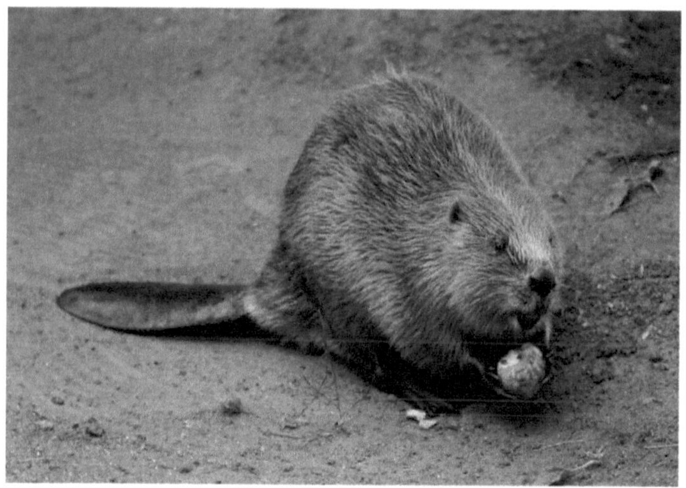

Figure 23. A beaver [5].

It is of interest for skin cures: against skin allergies, eczema (an antimicrobial antifungal, against chronic atopic dermatitis, from its medical name), it soothes redness and itching (an anti-inflammatory), and dermal dryness (a humectant: reduces oxidative stress and helps a dermatological preparation retain moisture in the skin), and it is potentially a healing agent [6].

Its more or less inexpensive price and environmental friendliness, which are attractive features, give it greater value, despite its non-domestibility.

It can be applied to the skin in oily form, or more recently, as a matrix in a biodegradable, biocompatible nanocomposite film, in dressings functionalized with chitosan (CS) and modified ZnO nanoparticles (NPs). All the characteristics of the bio-nanocomposite dressings, seemed to improve and approach commercial dressing standards, by increasing the filling of castor oil polymer films, with CS-ZnO nanoparticles. Pure castor oil polymer films (the only component) disintegrated easily, compared with those reinforced with CS-ZnO NPs.

Castor oil/chitosan and zinc oxide nanoparticle bionanocomposite films were found to be more biocidal, as the reinforcement of the castor oil polymer matrix by CS-ZnO nanoparticles increased. On the other hand, a biocidal affinity was noted against *Staphylococcus aureus*, and *Micrococcus luteus* compared to *Escherichia coli*, indicating the antibacterial power against Gram-positive

104

bacteria, of the bionanocomposite film.

However, it is accepted that the minimum inhibitory concentrations of CS-ZnO NPs in the reinforced films must be respected in order not to cause cytotoxic incompatibility with human skin, and it is also accepted that the addition of CS-ZnO NPs reinforcements to castor oil polymer films is carried out to ensure faster healing, which cannot be achieved with castor oil alone, or with gauze dressings [2].

Important information:

Castor oil, a biosourced polymer, currently accounts for the world's largest tonnage of biopolymer production, at over 500,000 tonnes per year [7]. Castor oil is an anionic surfactant, applied in pharmacology and cosmetology, and the only oil that is completely miscible with water, by the addition of sulfuric acid, so it is known as sulfonated castor oil, or otherwise called sulfated castor oil [8].

References

1. https://fr.wikipedia.org/wiki/Huile_de_ricin.

2. Díez-Pascual, A.M.; Díez-Vicente, A.L.. Wound Healing Bionanocomposites Based on Castor Oil Polymeric Films Reinforced with Chitosan-Modified ZnO Nanoparticles. Biomacromolecules 2015, 16, 2631-2644.

3. https://guide-huiledericin.fr/quest-ce-que-lhuile-de-castor.

h   ttps://www.paruvendu.fr/annonces/maison-jardin/graines-de-ricin--chauffailles- 71170/1260934188A1KBMAJA000: [4].

5. https://www.vigoenfotos.com/es/vigo/zoo/castor?p=2.

6. https://www.typology.com/carnet/l-huile-de-ricin-pour-soigner-l-eczema.

7. How to make polyamides from castor oil? www.mediachimie.org.

8. https://www.atamanchemicals.com/sulfonated-castor-oil_u25222/?lang=FR.

II.9.2. **Polyvinyl Alcohol (PVA)**

PVA is a synthetic, water-soluble polymer, acting as a thickener, or stabilizer, of polymerization [1], and at the same time it is an adsorbent of metals, even heavy ones, and cross-links with anionic and cationic molecules, thanks to the abundance of hydroxyl ($^-$OH) and acetate ($^-$O-CO-CH3) groups resident on PVA polymer chains. PVA enhances adsorption to the chitosan matrix (for stable delivery of proteins and active ingredients) [2].

During the freeze-thawing process, polysaccharides can easily bind to polyvinyl (alcohol), thanks to the large number of polar carboxyl and hydroxyl groups, giving rise to hydrogen bonds that form a simple 3D structure. The freeze-thawing process, with cross-linking by polyvinyl (alcohol) for a specific purpose, creates a biocompatible supramolecular network with a desirable rubbery and elastic nature, while also being non-toxic and non-carcinogenic. PVA, was interpenetrated with chitosan and zinc oxide nanoparticles, by the freeze-thaw method. The response surface methodology, modeled in 3D, the bionanocomposite hydrogels obtained, according to the essential process parameters:

- Defrosting time and temperature.

- Number of freeze-thaw cycles.

The variables they influence are :

- Water vapour transmission rate (WVTR).

- Porosity.

- absorption of wound exudates.

- Gel content: predefined intrinsic substrate concentrations, or sometimes the degree of swelling % H2O in the swollen, cross-linked network.

At room temperature and standard pressure, the resulting interpenetrating network was either, let's say, superconducting [3], ideal for full propagation of electrostatic Van der Vaals forces of attraction, and a medium where coagulum impurities, produced by electrostatic repulsion, linked to the NPs' surface charges, are virtually eliminated [3] [4]. If the claims are true, this antiseptic, healing nanocomposite biogel will transform the field from electricity and electronics to biomedicine [3].

References

1. https://en.wikipedia.org/wiki/Polyvinyl_alcohol.

2. Mok, C.F.; Ching, Y.C.; Muhamad,F.; Azuan Abu Osman, N.; Dai Hai, N.; Rosmani Hassan, C.. Adsorption of Dyes Using Poly(vinyl alcohol) (PVA) and PVA-Based Polymer Composite Adsorbents: A Review. Journal of Polymers and the Environment. Springer Science+Business Media, LLC, part of Springer Nature 2020.

3. Khorasani, M.T.; Joorabloo, A.; Adelib, H.; Mansoori-Moghadam, Z.; Moghaddam, A.. Design and optimization of process parameters of polyvinyl (alcohol)/ chitosan/nano zinc oxide hydrogels as wound healing materials. Carbohydrate Polymers 207 (2019) 542-554.

4. Water treatment - Coagulation-flocculation generalities - Degremont® (suezwaterhandbook.com).

Conclusion Chapter 9

For patches containing bionanocomposite functionalization films, the parameters to be analyzed for validation are as follows:

- Morphology (roughness and uniform distribution).
- Structure (degree of porosity).
- Thermal stability.
- Water absorption (hydrophilicity to dry exudates).
- Water vapour transmission rate (problem of overly volatile compounds).
- Biodegradability.
- Cytocompatibility.
- Mechanical properties (resistance to breaking point, tensile strength).
- Viscoelastic properties (flexibility and elasticity).
- Antibacterial properties and barrier and healing efficacy.

Dressings are tested against dry, simulated body fluid environments.

The aim is that the more the polymer films of functionalized topical dressings are in a moist atmosphere, the more flexible and supple they should become on the lesion, without disintegrating. Flexibility depends primarily on the amount of water absorbed by the bionanocomposite films in their initial states, as water plasticizes rapidly [1]. The porous nature of hydrogel dressings, and projectively that of film dressings, provides a suitable environment similar to the extracellular matrix (ECM), enabling good cell adhesion and growth, favoring the absorption of wound exudates. So, the higher the porosity of the products, the better the performance of the systems available as dressings. In addition, gel content determines the content of cross-linked polymer chains in the structure of hydrogels, affecting their strength and flexibility.

The method of modeling response surfaces is a revolutionary discovery that will transform the fields of biomedical electricity and electronics. While the use of the freeze-thaw method in the synthesis of hydrogels is a better alternative to the use of a chemical cross-linker, which often causes a toxic effect on the skin and represents a hazard in pharmaceutical waste, it also leads to a more fragile hydrogel structure, compared with the long-term stability of physical hydrogels obtained by the Freeze-Thawing process [2].

References

1. Diez-Pascual, A.M.; Diez-Vicente, A.L.. Wound Healing

Bionanocomposites Based on Castor Oil Polymeric Films Reinforced with Chitosan-Modified ZnO Nanoparticles. Biomacromolecules 2015, 16, 2631-2644.

2. Khorasani, M.T.; Joorabloo, A.; Adelib, H.; Mansoori-Moghadam, Z.; Moghaddam, A.. Design and optimization of process parameters of polyvinyl (alcohol)/ chitosan/nano zinc oxide hydrogels as wound healing materials. Carbohydrate Polymers 207 (2019) 542-554.

Chapter 10: How to update my knowledge of topical bionanocomposites

Foreword "Chapter 10

You may find this chapter interesting, dear readers, if you want to keep up to date with the latest scientific research on the subject of antiseptic bionanocomposites. You'll get the most important general ideas on a subject that captivates the attention of today's passionate medical students.

Les Pansements Films :

Given its easy availability, relatively inexpensive price and environmental friendliness, beaver oil was used in a 2015 study as a matrix for wound-healing film dressings filled with modified CS-ZnO NPs (by adding NaOH and sonication). Among the analyses carried out on the dressings are their :

- Morphology (roughness...in short, for marketing purposes).

- Structure (to guarantee a better therapist effect).

- Thermal stability (for safe storage at outside temperatures).

- Hydrophilia (absorbing wound exudates).

- Biodegradability (to protect the environment).

- Cytocompatibility (minimal cytotoxicity).

- Barrier properties (watertightness of dressings).

- Viscoelastic properties (dressings that attach well and don't tear easily).

- Anti-bacterial properties.

As the concentration of CS-ZnO nanofillers NPs increases ↑ , in a biopansement matrix and plasticized by freeze-drying (sous-vide) :

- Hydrophilia increases ↑ (drying of wound exudates).

- Thermal stability increases ↑ (guaranteed shelf life) .

- Degree of porosity increases ↑ (better wound drying).

- Water vapor transmission rate (WVTR) increases ↑ (better wound hydration).

- Oxygen permeability increases ↑ (a well-ventilated wound) (Diez-Pascual; 2015).

References :

Diez-Pascual, A.M.; Diez-Vicente, A.L., (2015). Wound Healing Bionanocomposites Based on Castor Oil Polymeric Films Reinforced with Chitosan-Modified ZnO Nanoparticles, Biomac, 16, 2631-2644.

Recent advances in the nano-engineering of cellulose as a carrier of active ingredients or incorporated into medical devices.

Over the last decade, there has been a growing demand for the substitution of synthetic materials with platforms of natural origin, to minimize their undesirable footprints on biomedicine, the environment and ecosystems. Among natural materials, cellulose, the world's most abundant biopolymer with key properties such as biocompatibility, bio-renewability and durability, has received considerable attention. The hierarchical structure of cellulose fibers, the main constituents of the plant cell wall, has been nanoengineered and fused into blocky biomedical constructs, providing nanoscale infrastructure within pharmaceutical sub-works or devices, such as implants and surgical instruments, in nanomedicine. Microorganisms, such as certain types of bacteria, are another source of nanocelluloses known as nanocellulose bacteria (NCB), which benefit from high purity and crystallinity. Chemical and mechanical treatments of cellulose fibrils, made up of alternating crystalline and amorphous regions, produce cellulose nanocrystals (CNC), hairy cellulose nanocrystals (Hairy CNC) and cellulose nanofibrils (CNF), with dimensions ranging from a few nanometers to several microns. Cellulose nanocrystals and nanofibrils can easily bind to drugs, proteins and nanoparticles via physical interactions, or be chemically modified to covalently accommodate cargoes. Surface engineering properties, such as chemical functionality, charge, surface area, crystallinity and hydrophilicity, play a central role in controlling cargo loading/rejection capacity and rate, stability, toxicity, immunogenicity and biodegradation of nanocellulose-based delivery platforms. This review provides an overview of recent advances in the nano-engineering of cellulose crystals and fibrils to develop vehicles, encompassing colloidal nanoparticles, hydrogels, aerogels, films, coatings, capsules and membranes, for the delivery of a wide range of bioactive cargoes, such as chemotherapy (anti-cancer) drugs, anti-inflammatory agents, antibacterial and probiotic compounds (antibiotics of bacterial or yeast origin, in short made from microorganisms naturally present in the human body, useful as antidiarrheals, and to treat certain infections) (Sheikhi ; 2018).

Mots-Clés Du Manuscrit (Sheikhi; 2018) :

Nanocellulose; Cellulose nanocrystals; Hairy nanocellulose; Bacterial cellulose; Cellulose nanofibrils; Drug delivery; Wound healing; Cancer treatment.

References :

Amir Sheikhi, Joel Hayashi, James Eichenbaum, Mark Gutin, Nicole Kuntjoro, Danial Khorsandi, Ali Khademhosseini, Recent advances in nanoengineering cellulose for cargo delivery. Corel (2018), https://doi.org/10.1016/j.jconrel.2018.11.024.

The Application of Biopolymer Hydrogel Products in Tissue Engineering

Decades have passed since the concept of tissue engineering was first put forward, and in recent years it has developed rapidly. Tissue substitutes, for artificial blood vessels, skin, bone and heart repair, have been extensively studied not only in the field of research, but also in clinical cases. For tissue engineering, scaffolds, also known as structural composites or block composites, are an indispensable component, which have also seen a shift from synthetic to natural materials with good biocompatibility. On the other hand, hydrogels prepared from natural polymers have properties similar to those of the ecosystem environment, and have the advantage of promoting cell adhesion, proliferation and targeting. These medical bionanocomposites, in their various forms, thanks to their biocompatibility, biodegradability and porosity, are commonly applied in cell culture neurogenesis, cardiac repair (pacemaker or = pacemaker or = cardiac battery) and bone and cartilage reconstruction (prostheses). Although a great deal of research has been carried out into tissue-engineered scaffolds, few have been commercialized, even after overcoming the drawback of insufficient mechanical properties. Since the human body is delicate, balancing the strength of scaffolds with the rate of tissue formation is one of the most difficult problems to solve, limiting their uses in the present. In addition, ensuring blood and tissue biocompatibility, to overcome rejection by the immune system, also requires a large number of clinical experiments. With the advent of three-dimensional printing technology, and artificial intelligence, the manufacture of bio-hydrogels, would be more practical and intelligent, and could overcome the problems of existing medical devices, such as implants and prostheses...and this would benefit a greater number of patients, with organ damage (Yang; 2020).

References :

Yang, J.; Sun, X.; Zhang, Y.; Chen, Y.; (2020). The application of natural polymer based hydrogels in tissue engineering. Hydrogels Based on Natural Polymers, Chapter 10 (273-307).

New Asymmetric Chitosan-Polyvinylpyrrolidone-Nanocellulose Dressings "CS-PVP-NC Systems": In Vitro and In Vivo Evaluation :

A wound can be defined as an acute injury, which damages the dermis of the skin and disrupts the normal anatomical (body) relationship of tissues due to an accident or suture. Wound healing is a multifactorial, physiological and complicated process, and generally needs to be covered by a dressing immediately after damage, as complications associated with wounds include infection, deformity, scar tissue proliferation and bleeding. Several dressing products are commercially available in the form of: non-adherent dressings, emollient dressings, film dressings, hydrocolloids, hydrogels, hydrofibers, foam dressings, antimicrobial dressings, charcoal dressings and composite dressings. In recent years, wound healing based on biopolymer dressings has been widely used, such as the abundant natural chitosan, due to its non-toxic character, and its biocompatible, biodegradable, moisturizing properties. What's more, it's readily available.

Chitosan has all the ideal properties for accelerating the wound-healing process. Chitosan is a 3-1,4-linked polymer of glucosamine (2-amino-2-deoxy-3-D-glucose) and smaller amounts of N-acetyl glucosamine. It is derived from chitin (poly-N-acetyl glucosamine), the second most abundant biopolymer after cellulose. Chitosan is a unique natural polymer with properties such as biocompatibility and biodegradability, all of which derive from the presence of the primary amine group on the backbone of its structure. It can be used in the treatment of wounds and burns due to its intrinsic antimicrobial property and hemostatic potential. A great deal of research in this field concludes that chitosan remains a suitable treatment for wounds and burns.

However, the application of chitosan can be limited by its poor mechanical properties, and the loss of its structural integrity. To overcome these drawbacks, chitosan is blended with synthetic polymers to broaden its range of applications. Biopolymer blending, too, is one of the most effective methods of creating new biomaterials with the desired properties. Chitosan/PVP blends have been attracting interest over the past decade, as their properties can be tailored to suit desirable needs and applications.

Polyvinylpyrrolidone (PVP), also known as polyvidone or povidone, is a synthetic, water-soluble, biocompatible polymer used for many biomedical applications, including wound dressings, and represents the main component in the development of temporary skin coverings, due to its transparency. PVP combines with iodine to form an antiseptic povidone-iodine solution with excellent disinfectant properties that are used for many medical purposes. However, skin disinfection with povidone-iodine is less common than for disinfecting surgical instruments, due to its undesirable effects on the skin, such as the risk of irritability, burns and severe allergic reactions in some patients. Several studies have reported the compatibility of chitosan and PVP, as they are easily miscible with each other.

The introduction of nanotechnology is one of the most important recent advances.

In this field, effective modification of blends is achieved to improve the properties of biopolymers, thus broadening their fields of application. Nanocellulose (NC) is a cellulose derivative composed of a network of nano-sized fibers, which has attracted a great deal of attention and interest in recent decades, due to its value-added biomedical applications. In recent years, considerable attention has been paid to nanocellulose-based materials, and their applications in wound dressing. Nanocellulose is suitable for wound dressing applications, as it possesses a number of interesting features, including its fine structure, high specific surface area, good mechanical and rheological properties, barrier properties, lack of toxicity and biocompatibility. Recently, several studies have investigated the potential of ternary polymer blends in biomedical applications.

Today, many polymers, including natural materials, synthetic materials and combinations of both, are combined with nanoparticles to produce nanocomposites for biomedical applications.

In conclusion, a new Chitosan-PVP-Nanocellulose composite dressing with symmetrical and asymmetrical structures modified by a thin stearic acid coating has been successfully prepared for application in wound healing. Thanks to the stearic acid coating, we have produced hydrophobic microporous surfaces, while the uncoated side is a macroporous hydrophilic surface. TEM and SEM proved its homogeneity and high porosity.

Symmetrical and asymmetrical Chitosan-Poly(vinylpyrrolidone)-nanocellulose bionanocomposite wound-healing dressings showed almost similar physicochemical properties, such as mechanical properties, high swelling capacity, moderate moisturizing properties and oxygen permeability (the process of coating dressings with stearic acid, seems to be optional, without cytotoxic and antibacterial analyses). The best properties in terms of physiological biocompatibility and antibacterial capacity are produced by asymmetrical dressings containing no more than 3% nanocellulose in the polymer blend Chitosan-Poly(Vinylpyrrolidone)-nanocellulose, with stearic acid. The in vivo wound-healing study showed that asymmetric dressings (temporary biological wound-healing agents) with precisely this concentration of nanocellulose biopolymers healed wounds faster than control wounds (without any treatment, and without nanocellulose, or with 5% nanocellulose). However, complete wound closure was expected by day 21eme . This can be seen by visual histological analysis (related to histology, the study of the formation of living tissue), in excellent re-epithelialization and dense collagen formation. This bionanocomposite dressing coated by the hydrophobic side of stearic acid, with 3% nanocellulose, could be tried as a wound dressing material, but tested on animals smaller or larger than albino rats, for application to humans (Poonguzhali; 2018).

References :

Poonguzhali, R.; Khaleel Basha, S.; Sugantha Kumari, V.; (2018). Novel asymmetric chitosan/PVP/nanocellulose wound dressing: In vitro and in vivo evaluation. BIOMAC 9127.

New Trends in Conductive Polymer Nanocomposites and Bionanocomposites:

Nanotechnological advances have shed light on the evolution of nanocomposites at the nanoscale. Intrinsic conductive polymers have been widely investigated due to intrinsically mysterious electronic technologies, as well as reduction-oxidation attributes and diverse potential uses in many fields.

With the emergence of nanotechnology, the manufacture of multifunctional conductive polymer nanocomposites (CPNCs) has attracted a great deal of attention in order to improve and multiply their behavior. CPNCs are composed of one or more components, such as graphene, graphite oxide, chalcogenides, graphene nanoplatelets (CNTs), metals, metal oxides, conductive or insulating polymers, biological entities, metal phthalocyanines, porphyrins, and other nanomaterials...

Applications for CPNCs include biological and chemical sensors, electronic nanodevices, electromagnetic interference (EMI) shielding, catalysis and electrocatalysis, energy, microwave absorption, electrorheological (ER) fluids, and biomedicine. The cumulative advantages of CPNCs (conductive polymers nanocomposites) over parent CPs (conductive polymers) have been clearly demonstrated.

Many designs and fabrications of conductive polymer nanomaterials, have emerged, especially CPs in conjunction with materials such as metals, metal oxides, chalcogenides, carbon derivatives, with variable architectural arrangement and oriented multi-component systems. Different synthesis methods result in variable architectural arrangements and nanocomposite dimensions for versatile applications. Thanks to their excellent electronic qualities, CPNCs can be widely explored for use in cardiac batteries, for example. In addition, they are chemically and biologically high-precision sensors. Conductive polymer nanocomposites protect against electromagnetic waves, corrosion, spark ignition and discharge explosions. When it comes to the design and synthesis of virgin (parent) conductive polymers, the major challenges are to manipulate the inherent electrical conductivity, and to vary the geometric and morphological arrangements of the components, in order to better functionalize these materials. Pure conductive polymers are therefore deficient in terms of throughput and cycle time for biosensors (detectors of complementary DNA, proteins, antigens, antibodies or diseases, also known as biosensors or biochips = medical devices measuring just a few square centimetres). New synthetic routes and alignment procedures capable of facilitating the large-scale manufacture of nanomaterials, based on conductive polymers, need to be provided. Essentially, we should propose methods for characterizing and controlling the crystalline-amorphous architectural distribution of conductive polymers incorporated into nanocomposites (Idumah; 2021).

References :

Idumah, C.I. ; (2021). Review: Novel trends in conductive polymeric nanocomposites, and bionanocomposites. Synthetic Metals, 273 (2021) 116674.

GENERAL CONCLUSION

There will be many more scientific publications on bionanocomposites in the future, and the diversification of raw materials of natural origin will ensure the balance of our ecosystem.

The study we've carried out follows the third law enunciated by Issac Newton in 1687, i.e. the fact of understanding certain phenomena by understanding their opposite phenomena: the preformulation of a chemical bionanocomposite hydrogel must pass through the mastery of the preformulation of the physical bionanocomposite hydrogel.

Our manipulations are based on two research articles: Kozicki et al. (2016) / Sun et al. (2015), after reading in great detail, over a period of 3 years, without characterization by physico-chemical analysis devices, i.e. by visual and tactile analysis.

But our visual and tactile analysis was enhanced by careful reading of several original works and literature, as well as by the prior knowledge of our supervisors, before and during the manipulations. In addition to the bibliographical verification of the results, in the form of a well-studied statistical analysis, after the manipulations.

We have left it up to the reader to choose the best method for preparing the CS/ Nano Ag antiseptic hydrogel, as each method has its own advantages and disadvantages. While the results of the method of Kozicki et al. (2016), are characterized by an above-average sensitivity, the method of Sun et al. (2015), was characterized by the high specificity of the results.

The reaction mechanism proposed in this thesis is also theoretical, and H-bonds have been neglected, but another more detailed mechanism is to be worked out by subsequent researchers. Although very enriching, and important in the theme of this thesis, re-explanations, have been avoided in the general conclusion of the book. We have chosen not to deal with the information in Chapters 5, 6, 7, 8 and 9 or 10 on this page of the thesis. Note that this method of writing is more reasonable, in a book, in process engineering, compared to theses letters and languages.

THESIS SUMMARY "RESEARCH ON THERAPEUTIC BIONANOCOMPOSITES

The aim of this scientific work is to formulate a bionanocomposite with topical antiseptic efficacy.

It has been noted that theses talking solely about bionanocomposites are rare, so this book can be a reference on chitosan, itself, or on chitosan bionanocomposite hydrogels, functionalized with silver nitrate and stabilized by sodium hydroxide. It highlights the importance of supramolecular complexation of chitosan particles, and includes the reaction mechanism that occurs between chitosan monomers, and acetic acid molecules in aqueous media, with a specific technique that enables Nano chitosans to be obtained. In addition, the definition of bionanocomposite hydrogels was well explained.

Key words :

Antimicrobial agent.

Bionanocomposite.

Biopolymer.

Metallic nanoparticles.

Pharmaceutical Textile (Bionanocomposite Hydrogel has been manufactured for given conditions).

ملخص أطروحة البحث عن المركبات الحيوية ذات الفضيلة العلاجية

ينصب اهتمام هذا العمل العلمي على صياغة مركب بيونانوكومبوزيت له فعالية مطهرة موضعية. لقد لوحظ أن الأطروحات التي تتحدث فقط عن المركبات الحيوية نادرة، لذلك يمكن أن يكون هذا الكتاب مرجعًا للكيتوزان، نفسه، أو على هيدروجيلات الكيتوزان ثنائية المركب، التي تعمل مع نترات الفضة وتستقر بواسطة هيدروكسيد الصوديوم. يسلط الضوء على أهمية التعقيد فوق الجزيئي لجزيئات الشيتوزان، ويتضمن آلية التفاعل التي تحدث بين مونومرات الكيتوزان وجزيئات حمض الأسيتيك في الوسط المائي، مع تقنية محددة تسمح بالحصول على نانو كيتوزان. بالإضافة إلى ذلك، تم شرح تعريف الهلاميات المائية ثنائية المركب بشكل جيد.

الكلمات الرئيسية:

عامل مضاد للميكروبات.	جزيئات نانوية معدنية.
مركب نانوي حيوي.	نسيج صيدلاني (تم تصنيع هيدروجيل نانوي حيوي).
بوليمر حيوي.	

ACKNOWLEDGEMENT

& DEDICATED

Thank You, Dear parents

Thank You, Dear teachers.

Cordially,

M. GANDI or called "Salima".

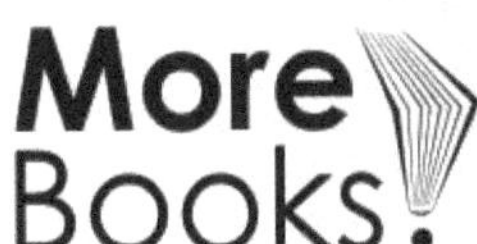

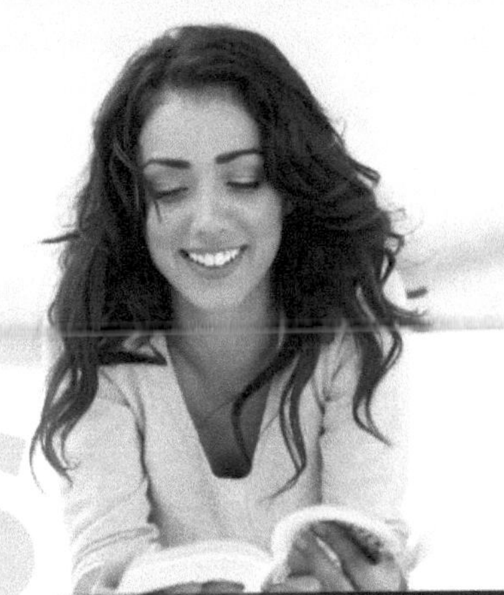

I want morebooks!

Buy your books fast and straightforward online - at one of world's fastest growing online book stores! Environmentally sound due to Print-on-Demand technologies.

Buy your books online at
www.morebooks.shop

Kaufen Sie Ihre Bücher schnell und unkompliziert online – auf einer der am schnellsten wachsenden Buchhandelsplattformen weltweit! Dank Print-On-Demand umwelt- und ressourcenschonend produziert.

Bücher schneller online kaufen
www.morebooks.shop

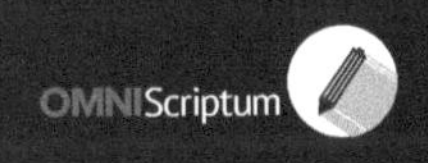

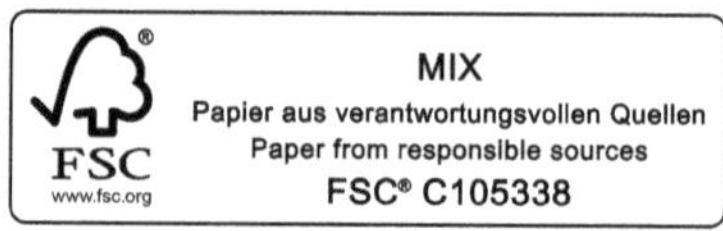

Printed by Books on Demand GmbH, Norderstedt / Germany